The Governance Factor

33 Keys to Success

in Healthcare

The Governance Factor

33 Keys to Success in Healthcare

ERROL L. BIGGS

Health Administration Press

ACHE MANAGEMENT SERIES

Your board, staff, or clients may also benefit from this book's insight. For more information
Your board, staff, or clients may also benefit from this book's insight. For more information
on quantity discounts, contact the Health Administration Press Marketing Manager at (312) 424-9470.

08   07   06   05   04   5   4   3   2   1

Library of Congress Cataloging-in-Publication Data

Biggs, Errol.
The governance factor: 33 keys to success in healthcare/by Errol L. Biggs
    p.cm.
Includes bibliographical references
ISBN 1-56793-213-4 (alk. paper)
1. Hospitals—Administration. 2. Hospital trustees. I. Title.

RA971.B57 2003
362.11'068—dc22

                          2003056615

The paper used in this publication meets the minimum requirements of American National Standard for Information Sciences—Permanence of Paper for Printed Library Materials, ANSI Z39.48-1984. ∞™

Acquisitions manager: Audrey Kaufman; Project manager: Cami Cacciatore; Layout editor: Amanda J. Karvelaitis; Cover design: Betsey Perez

Health Administration Press
A division of the Foundation of the
    American College of
    Healthcare Executives
1 North Franklin Street, Suite 1700
Chicago, IL 60606-4425
(312) 424-2800

Contents

This book is dedicated to Alison Knight Biggs,
truly a lovely lady,
whose husband I have the privilege to be.

PREFACE

THE WORK OF a healthcare organization board is challenging even in the best of times. Being a hospital board member today is much more difficult than it was just five years ago. However, in these turbulent times, we are fortunate to still have sincere, well-meaning individuals willing to take on this formidable task. It is important to support them in this work, whether they are just getting started or are seasoned members encountering new ideas or challenges to old ones.

Although I have worked with many boards of directors throughout my career in the healthcare industry, I am continuously intrigued by how boards of like-sized hospitals from like-sized communities can vary so much in how efficiently they function. Certainly, no individual goes on a board to be ineffective. One problem seems to be that many otherwise very competent individuals have never received job descriptions or an effective orientation session, and they simply don't know their roles and responsibilities as productive healthcare board members.

This book then is designed so that it can be used by both new and experienced board members. It provides a focus on 33 important questions—keys, if you will—relating to board structure and function and board members' responsibilities. The identification of these questions, and the development of the answers, actually began during the several years I spent running hospitals and later attending eight to ten management-contract hospital board meetings a month. The work has been further advanced from my subsequent years of experience serving on boards, working and interacting with boards, teaching graduate students about governance, and consulting for and doing research about boards.

Most recently, I conducted a quick and random survey of hospital CEOs in the United States. Although the 12 percent return was lower than I anticipated (perhaps an indication of the full schedules these individuals have), the survey was useful in confirming how the healthcare industry is paying attention to governance issues. The lists below compare the results of this survey with the results of a similar survey done with CEOs of public companies. Both groups were asked to identify two or three main issues they felt their boards were or should be addressing, and the tabulation of the top ten is as follows:

Hospital CEOs
1. Financial survival and generation of capital (27%)
2. Strategic planning (25%)
3. Conflict of interest among board members (17%)
4. Quality-of-care oversight (15%)
5. Board evaluation and education (10%)
6. Community relations and needs (8%)
7. Accomplishing the organization's mission and vision (8%)
8. Physician relations (retention and recruitment) (7%)
9. Term and age limits for board members (6%)
10. Board selection process (5%)

Public Company CEOs
1. Corporate performance (28%)
2. CEO successsion (25%)
3. Strategic planning (15%)
4. Corporate governance (10%)
5. Board-CEO relations (6%)
6. Mergers and acquisitions (5%)
7. Executive compensation (3%)
8. Owner-shareholder relations (2%)
9. Relations with other constituencies (2%)
10. Risk-management programs (2%)

Both groups are obviously interested in the overall topic of governance and in attending to those key areas they feel will make their boards effective for the benefit of the organization. Regardless of tax status, we all seem to be in a very similar boat.

The last question in the hospital survey asked the CEOs, "If you could list just one question a board should ask itself in a self-assessment survey, what would the question be?" The top five questions included the following:

1. Is the board effective in accomplishing its mission?
2. Does each board member understand his or her role and responsibilities?
3. Does each board member understand the mission and make decisions that are in the best interest of the community?
4. Does each board member understand the healthcare industry?
5. Does the board understand the difference between governance functions and management functions?

These results confirmed that the type of information I had planned to include in this book would be useful for those involved in healthcare organization governance. As it is structured, the book can be perused in sections, allowing the reader to go to specific areas of interest or need, or it can be considered as a whole. The goal was to present information in a format that would be helpful regardless of the expertise of anyone using it.

I would like to thank some groups and individuals who were very helpful in developing several areas of the book: Kenneth Bopp, PH.D. (clinical professor, director, Health Management & Informatics Group, University of Missouri, Columbia); Donna Marshall (executive director, Colorado Business Group on Health, Denver); Bruce Neumann, PH.D. (professor of accounting and health management, University of Colorado at Denver); Gregory Piche (partner, Holland & Hart, Denver, Colorado); Michael Pugh (principal, Pugh Ettinger McCarthy Associates, LLC, Pueblo, Colorado); Larry Tyler (president, Tyler & Company, Atlanta, Georgia); Cathy Barry-Ipema (chief communications officer, Joint Commission on Accreditation of Healthcare Organizations, Oakbrook Terrace, Illinois); and Alison K. Biggs, MSHA, RN.

CHAPTER ONE

Basic Responsibilities of a Board and Its Members

What Are the Main Responsibilities of the Governing Board?

...or, What Are We Supposed to Be Doing?

While some may feel it is obvious that "the board runs the show," that kind of simplistic approach ignores the complexity of reality. Without a knowledge of and attention to the basic components of a board's reason for being, a board inadvertently abdicates its responsibilities.

The board has the responsibility for envisioning, formulating, and amending the organization's mission, vision, and goals

It is the board's responsibility to map the hospital's course through the establishment and periodic review of the hospital's mission, vision, and goals. As has frequently been said, "If you don't know where you are going, any road will take you there."

Without a clear understanding and agreement of what the organization wants to accomplish (the mission), how it wants to accomplish it (the goals), and where it wants to be in the future (the vision), a board can wander countless roads, never knowing when it has accomplished something of value or even what is valued. Strategic planning (discussed later in this chapter) is a function of the board that ties these three components together.

Once the mission, vision, and goals are established and a strategic plan is developed, the board will then be able to reach its decisions accordingly. However, experience has shown that board members frequently are not really aware of the hospital's mission.

The simple act of putting the mission statement at the top of the agenda for every board meeting can save time and unnecessary discussion. If board members can readily see the mission statement, their course of action will be more obvious. Some agenda items may even be dispensed with quickly if it is obvious they are not part of the mission.

To focus the entire organization on the mission statement, it should be printed clearly on the back of all business cards and at the top of agendas for any hospital-related meetings of the board, employees, medical staff, or volunteers.

The board has the responsibility for ensuring a high level of executive management performance (Chapter Two)

When dealing with the organization's staff, the board should concentrate on the only employee who reports directly to the board—the chief executive officer (CEO). Although the chief operating officer, chief financial officer, chief nursing officer, medical director, and any vice presidents are very important people in making the organization a success, the board does not need to concern itself with any of these individuals. Many boards have difficulty, particularly in smaller communities where everyone tends to know each other, staying focused on the CEO; however, it is important for that focus to remain clear. The board does not evaluate anyone but the CEO, does not hire anyone but the CEO, does not set goals and objectives for anyone except the CEO, and does not replace anyone but the CEO. CEO succession planning is an important component of the latter, ensuring that the organization does not flounder during any time of transition from one CEO to a successor.

The board has the ultimate responsibility for ensuring the quality of patient care (Chapter Three)

The board may and should delegate the design, implementation, and measurement of the quality of care provided in the hospital to administration and the medical staff. However, the board is legally and ultimately responsible for ensuring quality care is available and provided to patients. As such, the board needs to be comfortable that the systems are in place to make that assurance, and it needs to see quality indicators that allow a lay board member to understand how high the hospital's quality is compared to similar organizations (benchmarking).

There are many quality outcome indicators: hospital-acquired infections; surgical wound infections; neonatal mortality; inpatient mortality; Cesarean-section rate; unplanned readmissions to the hospital; unplanned returns to the operating room; pressure ulcers (bed sores); patient falls; nurse hours per patient day; patient satisfaction with pain management; and overall patient satisfaction, just to name a few. The board, through its quality committee, should develop dashboard indicators to alert it to quality outcome measurements the board would not find acceptable.

Effective boards raise the importance of quality to equal or surpass that of finance. This sends a very clear message to administration, the medical staff, nursing staff, and others. These boards strive to run hospitals that benchmark very well in all areas of quality measurement.

The board has the ultimate responsibility for ensuring the organization's financial health (Chapter Four)

Financial health and high quality are explicitly intertwined. Most board members feel a little more comfortable in reviewing financial statements than quality indicators. However, in many instances, experienced business people somehow have a different view of what financial health means in a nonprofit hospital. Some nonprofit boards think nonprofit means not too much black ink, nor too much red ink, but "pink" ink—a kind of a break-even mentality.

A recently completed nationwide study (Biggs 2002) asked hospital CEOs what issues boards should be addressing. Response indicated the number one issue was how the hospital was going to survive financially and how the hospital was going to generate sufficient capital to replace equipment and facilities.

Boards must understand how important it is to have excess revenue over expense at least equal to the cost of capital. For example, if the board is to keep the hospital's equipment up-to-date or replace antiquated or inefficient buildings structures, it is imperative to have enough revenue/profit available to accomplish these things. As a faculty member from the University of Colorado at Denver, Dr. Leland Kaiser (1983) has said, "It is virtuous to *help* the poor; it is not virtuous to *be* poor!" A hospital is a business and must have excess revenue over expense to continue to provide quality care.

Increasingly hospital boards are being expected to assume some responsibility for their community's health (Chapter Five)

While the responsibility for a community's health is a somewhat recent idea, many hospitals are now expected to more proactively assess and address the health status of their communities. It is the board's role to determine how this should be done within the organization's resources.

The board must assume responsibility for itself (Chapter Six)

The board has a responsibility for taking care of itself, including, at a minimum, establishing an effective orientation program for new members; a self-assessment process, which is conducted at least every two to three years; a continuing education program for all members, including subscriptions to magazines such as *Trustee*; and up-to-date job descriptions for all members and officers. Job descriptions are perhaps the most important of these. If new board members are given an up-to-date job description (see Appendix 3) by the board chair, there will be much less confusion about the role of the board, and the new members' specific roles on that board.

What is the Role of the Board in Strategic Planning?

...or, Which Way Do We Go?

In recent years, strategic planning is something boards of both private non-profit and public companies are saying is an important function. The National Association of Corporate Directors (NACD) conducts biennial surveys concerning board attitudes and practices. Their 2001–2002 survey of leading issues among public boards, which included non-CEO directors as well as CEO directors, found that strategic planning ranked third, behind corporate performance and CEO succession (NACD 2001). NACD also works with Institutional Shareholder Services (ISS), the world's largest proxy advisory firm. This relationship with ISS has enhanced their survey efforts, enabling NACD to incorporate data on the governance practices of over 5,000 public companies.

Similarly, in the study (Biggs 2002) that asked hospital CEOs what a board's main issues should be, strategic planning came in second, behind fiscal survival/capital generation. In today's turbulent environment, this similar emphasis on the importance of strategic planning is likely not a coincidence.

Boards should be actively engaged with management to ensure the appropriate development, execution, and modification of the healthcare organization's strategic plan, for several reasons. Advances in medical technology, competition from a hospital's medical staff, changing reimbursement patterns, consolidation in the healthcare industry, and stakeholder activism are all occurring with increasing rapidity. Organizations must respond to such changes with similar speed. Hospitals and healthcare organizations that do not have a carefully thought-out strategic plan are steering the organization in a dangerous direction.

Appropriate development of a strategic plan does not mean the board has to initially determine the organization's strategy or create the detailed strategic plan, as this is generally the responsibility of management. The role of management is to develop the organization's strategy, obtain board approval, develop plans to implement and communicate the strategy, routinely update the board on its execution, and propose changes in the strategy as needed. Management should also regularly send the board supplemental information relative to the performance of the organization, especially trends and uncertainties that may affect the implementation of the approved strategy.

The role of the board, on the other hand, is to evaluate the strategy proposed by management, challenge assumptions and analyses as necessary, approve the strategy, monitor its implementation, and encourage changes as events require. Simply put, management creates the organization's strategic plan, involving the full board in its development. With this understanding of the plan, the board will be able to intelligently monitor it and suggest needed changes and adjustments.

What Are the Basic Legal Duties a Director Should Remember?

...or, How Does a Board Stay Out of Trouble?

The duty of care

A director's duty of care relates to the director's responsibility to exercise appropriate diligence in making decisions as well as in overseeing management of the corporation. Generally, the duty of care requires directors to exercise reasonable care in the execution of their responsibilities, doing what a reasonable person would do in the same situation with the same information. The effect of this duty is to afford directors protection from liability for taking actions that they believe are in the best interests of the corporation, so long as there is some rational basis for their decisions and no conflicting interest is involved.

The duty of care rule also indicates that a director can rely on information, opinions, reports, or statements prepared by officers, employees, legal counsel, and committees provided the director acts in good faith—that is, has no knowledge that his or her actions are inappropriate. In meeting their duty of care, directors must be willing to make the appropriate time commitment for regular attendance at meetings, must stay informed about the issues before the board, and must be willing to ask the right questions during deliberations.

The duty of loyalty

The director owes loyalty to the organization and its stakeholders. The duty of loyalty requires a director to exercise authority in good faith, in the best interests of the corporation, and not in the director's own interest or the interest of another person (such as a family member) or another organization with which the director is associated. A director should not use the director's corporate position to make a personal profit or gain or for other personal advantage.

The duty of loyalty has some specific applications:

1. *Conflict of interest.* Each director should be alert and sensitive to any interest he or she may have that might be considered to conflict with the best interests of the corporation. Directors may not enter into contracts with the organization without full disclosure and approval. (See Appendix 1 for a sample conflict of interest policy and Appendix 2 for a sample conflict of interest disclosure statement.)
2. *Corporate opportunity.* The duty of loyalty generally requires a director to not undertake a business opportunity, if it is related to the business of the corporation, without first making the opportunity available to the corporation. To open a business in competition with the hospital would indeed be considered bad form. Whether such an opportunity should first be offered to the corporation will depend on the correlation of the opportunity to the corporation's existing business, the circumstances in which the director became aware of the opportunity, the degree of interest the corporation has in the opportunity, and the reasonableness of the basis for the corporation to expect that the director should make the opportunity available to the corporation.

The duty of obedience

Directors should not exceed their delegated authority or direct the organization beyond its purpose or mission as set forth by the articles of incorporation, bylaws, or constitution. Such actions violate the trust invested by those who support the organization and, in nonprofit organizations, could imperil their tax-exempt status. Basically, the duty of obedience requires the director to obey all laws and support the mission and bylaws of the organization. Officers and directors of healthcare organizations continue to be named as defendants in lawsuits for acts of their organizations. Although some immunities have been provided by statute and most organizations have director's and officer's (D & O) insurance, directors are encouraged to pay special attention to the authority granted them by the organization and to not deviate from it without the permission required by the organization's operating documents.

What Are the Main Committees a Healthcare Organization Should Have?

...or, Who Does What?

Committees exist to help the board perform its duties and meet its responsibilities. There do not seem to be any strong and fast rules about the number of committees a healthcare organization board should have nor what they should be called. However, the last thing a board should do is have too many committees, requiring members to attend more meetings than necessary. Care should be taken to appoint only those standing committees necessary to handle ongoing matters. Ad hoc committees can be formed to deal with issues of short-term duration or to complete a specific task and then dissolve when that task is accomplished. All committees are established to help the process of governance, and there should not be committees add-ressing obvious management functions.

In addition to assisting the board in handling its work efficiently, committees can play another very useful role within the organization. As it is sometimes difficult to recruit talented people for board membership, it may be quite useful to appoint one or two individuals who are not on the board to certain committees as volunteers. This is an excellent way to determine if someone would make a good board member in the future and to interest that individual in such service.

In general, a healthcare organization needs the following committees on a standing basis to function effectively.

Executive committee

The executive committee, comprising those members enumerated in the bylaws, should meet only when the board cannot easily have a quorum present. If the executive committee meets on a regular basis, it sometimes becomes the board, and governance decisions start to be made solely by the committee, only to be rubber-stamped by the full board. Before long, the full board feels the executive committee is making the major decisions and members can lose interest and motivation, or come to resent the executive committee members entirely—not a healthy situation.

Some of the key functions performed by the executive committee include the following:

- providing advice to the board chair in the appointment of committees and committee chairs;
- serving as a sounding board for the CEO;
- assisting the chair in developing the governance goals and objectives for the coming year;
- determining CEO compensation; and
- directing the CEO evaluation process.

Planning committee

This committee may also be called the strategic planning committee, and it is responsible for helping the board to formulate policies and develop goals and objectives and for determining in what strategic direction the organization is headed. Some of its specific duties include the following:

- developing and recommending the strategic plan for the organization;
- developing mechanisms to monitor this plan on a regular basis;
- occasionally completing an analysis of key stakeholders, which includes their interests and expectations;
- reviewing proposals submitted by management for board recommendation; and
- reviewing community health needs that should be incorporated in the planning process.

Quality and community health committee

This is an important committee whose work assures the board that the organization is providing quality care and addressing the health status of the community. At one time, this committee might have only involved itself in what went on inside the hospital's walls. However, in today's competitive environment, healthcare organizations have (and should) broaden their scope of involvement into the entire community; therefore, this committee must broaden its own scope accordingly.

With an expanded scope, this committee must be ensured an equal footing with the finance committee. When boards make it clear that the quality and community health committee is very important, it sends a message to the administration, medical staff, and others that quality really does matter and it is to be taken seriously.

Some specific duties of this committee include the following:

- making sure systems for measuring quality care in the organization are established, meaningful, and regularly reviewed;
- drafting policies regarding all aspects of quality, for review and adoption by the board;
- determining the community's health status and recommending actions to affect improvement;
- identifying potential collaborative relationships with other community health providers to enhance community health status; and
* diligently reviewing medical staff recommendations regarding appointment, reappointment, and privilege delineation of physicians and other practitioners.

Finance committee

The finance committee assists the board in maintaining and improving the financial integrity of the organization. Some of its specific functions include the following:

- drafting policies regarding finances for board review and adoption;
- developing kcy financial ratios to be utilized by the committee and specific ones for the board;

- reviewing the draft budget, including revenues, expenses, and capital expenditures for the coming year, and recommending its adoption to the board;
- completing a regular review of all board policies and decisions regarding finances; and
- performing other duties assigned by the board related to the organization's financial health.

Audit committee

In most healthcare organizations the audit function has been overseen by a subcommittee of the finance committee or by the finance committee as a whole. Current practice is evolving to have the audit committee report directly to the board.

The primary purposes of an audit committee are to foster and oversee strong financial reporting and controls and to help ensure the proper identification and management of risk—the array of forces that may have a negative impact on the organization's financial condition. The Sarbanes-Oxley Act (Public Law 107-204, July 30, 2002) and other regulatory changes now require more accountability for public companies and their boards. These new requirements do not yet apply to tax-exempt organizations, but they may soon be used as a standard for evaluating the performance of such organizations, especially those that issue tax-exempt bonds. Healthcare organizations should now consider appointing audit committees that report directly to the board and have the direct responsibility for the appointment, compensation, and oversight of the independent auditors, who must report directly to the audit committee.

Some specific functions of the audit committee include the following:

- recommending the selection and compensation of the external auditors to the board;
- overseeing the organization's internal audit function for the board;
- reviewing and being responsible for financial reporting and controls;
- reviewing and assessing the organization's business risk management process; and
- preapproving any nonauditing functions proposed by the external auditors.

The committee also is responsible for reviewing and approving the organization's code of ethical financial conduct and the definitions of significant conflicts of interest and related party transactions and the performance of both the external audit and the internal audit function.

Governance committee

The governance committee is the board committee charged with oversight of the board's organization and work processes and effectiveness.

Specific functions of the governance committee include the following:

- clarifying the duties and responsibilities of the board and its members;
- evaluating board structure and composition;
- nominating members of the board;
- monitoring policies and practices of the board;
- planning the annual board retreat; designing the board's new-member orientation process;
- directing the board's continuing education and development activities;
- arranging for the completion of the board's self-assessment process;
- analyzing the results of the self-assessment process;
- regularly reviewing all board policies and decisions regarding governance performance; and
- performing other duties related to governance assigned by the board.

What Are the Main Responsibilities of Individual Board Members?

...or, How Do I Fit in This Picture?

Board members frequently accept their roles with enthusiasm, tempered with hesitancy about being the new kid on the block. Those who have been around a while can either be very comfortable with their roles or become jaded and lax. Ideally, an individual board member will continually contribute to the advancement of the organization because they do the following:

1. *Understand the organization.* Board members need to understand the organization's mission, vision, goals, objectives, and bylaws and believe in them. Agreement with the mission is particularly important as it drives all decisions. If board members have the mission of the organization clearly in mind, most decisions will be easy to make.

2. *Develop a broad knowledge of the healthcare industry.* Board members are not necessarily expected to be experts on the healthcare industry, but they need to develop a broad knowledge of the industry and the trends in healthcare. The CEO can be very helpful in providing educational materials for this purpose. Members should also attend educational programs, read a few healthcare journals, and in general stay abreast of what is happening in the industry.

3. *Acquire a working knowledge.* Individual board members should acquire a fundamental knowledge about the functional areas related to committee assignments. For example, if a board member is assigned to the finance committee, the member should look for articles and materials related to finance committees of healthcare organizations. Again, the CEO can be very helpful in giving the board member materials to read and seminars to attend.

4. *Prepare.* Before meetings, board members should read all materials provided to them to allow them to deliberate intelligently during the meeting. Sometimes board members (particularly new ones) hesitate to ask questions or request information because they are intimidated by hospital jargon and medical terminology. A board member should *never* hesitate to ask questions or to indicate something is not understood. Board members should remember that serving on a hospital board is usually not their day job they cannot be expected to know what management, physicians, or more seasoned board members inherently know about hospital operations.

5. *Regularly attend meetings, and be on time.* Board members are expected to attend all board and committee meetings, arrive on time, and execute their assignments on time. In today's healthcare environment, a board cannot afford to have "letterhead" directors—people whose names appear on the organization's stationery but who do not attend meetings for whatever valid or invalid reasons. These people are also called "ornamental" directors and are essentially useless to the organization.

6. *Make a positive contribution.* A board member must make a positive contribution to board discussions, always keeping in mind the best interests of the corporation. This allows the board to reach sound conclusions and speak with one voice. A board is not a court or a legislative body; after adequate discussion, decisions should not be made on a 5-to-4 vote, and there should be no minority reports. It is totally inappropriate for an individual board member to indicate to someone outside of the board that a board decision was a bad one and he or she voted against it. The first time this occurs, it is the individual's fault and the board needs to make it clear this is not acceptable behavior. If there is a second time, the board must act to remove the individual from the board, or its effectiveness, teamwork, and credibility in the community will be severely damaged. In county and district hospitals where members come from varied sources, this can be difficult to accomplish, but the offending member must at least be counseled away from such destructive behavior.

7. *Don't dominate meetings.* Board members who dominate discussions, ignore the agenda, or digress to their own interests create problems for the board and for the CEO. An effective board chair will not allow this to happen, and other board members can also assist in keeping the meeting on track. Such behavior should be considered during the offending member's evaluation.

8. *Avoid rumors and gossip.* Board members should ask the CEO or the board president about rumors, gossip, or criticism of the hospital before drawing conclusions. This will allow the board and the CEO to work in tandem to handle incorrect information in an appropriate fashion.

9. *Avoid conflict of interest.* In today's turbulent environment, board members cannot give even the appearance of having a conflict of interest. In the nationwide study discussed earlier (Biggs 2002) that asked CEOs to identify the main issues boards should be addressing, conflict of interest was ranked third, ahead of quality and board evaluation. It is no longer acceptable for a board member with a conflict to simply abstain when a discussion or vote takes place on the conflicting issue.

   As an example, consider a hospital board in a town with five banks. Bill is a board member and also president of the bank where the hospital deposits its money. The finance committee has recommended the hospital should look at other banks to find a more competitive interest rate. The board chair says, "Bill, we're going to look at moving the hospital's money from your bank to another bank in town, so you better step out of the room and abstain from this discussion and vote because of your possible conflict of interest." Bill steps out of the room and after its discussion, the board decides to switch banks. The chair calls Bill back and says, "Well, Bill, we decided to move the hospital's money to XYZ bank. I hope you don't have a problem with that decision." What would be the likelihood of Bill being a cooperative, team-playing board member during the next few years? In another scenario, the rest of the board members could decide not to move the hospital's money out of loyalty to Bill rather than loyalty to the best interest of the hospital. This type of decision is also inappropriate.

The best solution then is to avoid placing an individual on the board who could have, or could have the appearance of having, a conflict of interest in the first place. Again, district or county hospitals have a particular difficulty in accomplishing this and must be extremely sensitive in this area. (Appendix 1 provides a sample conflict of interest policy, and Appendix 2 provides a sample conflict of interest disclosure statement.)

10. *Avoid interference in hospital operations.* This topic is one of particular importance and is a pitfall for many board members. The board needs to look down at the strategic future direction of the organization from "30,000 feet," where they can see the overall picture of where the organization is going without getting involved in the details of managing the process of getting there. If board members are functioning at the 5,000-foot level, they are too close to the management function and no longer able to stay out of the picture. Sometimes board members get involved in operations because the CEO has given the board management information instead of governance information. If the board receives governance information, it might just govern; but it will certainly try to manage if it receives detailed management information.

For example, governance information might include strategic planning specifics, information about possible mergers or major service changes, the organization's overall financial picture, or financial dashboard indicators. Management information would include such details as the color or design of a remodeled lobby, review of the points in a managed care contract, or financial records of individual department spending.

11. *Maintain hospital confidentiality.* Board members who share confidential information with outside parties present a real problem for the hospital and for the CEO. Certain board deliberations are most appropriately left in the boardroom, with publicity properly directed to final board action and not the discussions that led to that action. Board members should remember to check with the board president or the CEO if they have questions about how much and what type of information can be shared. It is the board's duty to keep confidential information inside the boardroom.

12. *Be a partner to the CEO.* Board members should act like partners and advisors to the CEO rather than as supervisors. The organization has a much better chance of success if the board and the CEO are functioning as a team. There will be a greater satisfaction level for both and a greater benefit to the organization. Board members also need to be honest and candid with the CEO. Discussing key issues behind the CEO's back leads to an unhealthy relationship between the CEO and the board. CEOs expect board members to be forthright and honest with them.

13. *Serve as a mentor/consultant.* An individual board member should be available to serve as a consultant and/or sounding board to the CEO and others in the organization when asked to do so on appropriate issues. Seasoned board members can also be very helpful to new board members as they learn their role in the organization and on the board.

14. *Be alert for new opportunities.* Board members should be alert for opportunities in the community that the hospital might address. As hospitals are increasingly being expected to assume some responsibility for their community's health, board members are in key positions to identify areas of need that the hospital might fill. Of course, by virtue of their occupations and positions, some board members have better opportunities for this than others, but all should be alert to this responsibility.

15. *Interpret the hospital to the community.* The individual board member should be a representative of the hospital, interpreting it and its functions to the community. While always remembering the need for confidentiality of certain information, and the need for the board to

speak with one voice, board members can be extremely influential in gathering support of all types for the hospital and its programs. As a side note, many hospitals lose or ignore their retired board members, but these individuals also can be very helpful if they continue their positive relationship with the organization. It requires very little effort on the hospital's part to keep retired board members informed and appropriately involved, and they can do wonders for the hospital in the community.

What Are the Responsibilities of the Board Chair?

...or, Do I Really Want to Take on This Job?

Eight basic responsibilities of a board chair are described below, and a sample job description for a board chair is provided in Appendix 3. Each chair will bring unique strengths and weaknesses to the role but should take care to ensure these responsibilities are carried out.

1. *Presides over all meetings of the board and executive committee.* The duties of the board and executive committee are enumerated in preceding sections. One duty of the chair is to run focused, creative, effective, and efficient board and executive committee meetings. Nothing is worse for a board than a chair who does not know how to preside over a meeting. If the chair does not possess these skills, he or she should learn them—fast.

2. *Designates board committees.* With the advice and consent of the executive committee, the chair designates board committees and committee chairs. The executive committee provides a good check and balance for the chair's selections.

3. *Serves as ex officio member of committees.* The chair serves as an ex officio member of all board committees. As such, the chair is not necessarily expected to attend these meetings, but may do so by virtue of the position.

4. *Serves as board's representative.* The chair serves as the board's primary representative to the community at large and to key stakeholder groups.

5. *Serves as a counselor to CEO.* The chair serves as a counselor to the CEO on matters of governance and board-CEO relations. There is possibly no more important function the chair fulfills than this one. The chair and the CEO must work together as a team, and the chair can be a tremendous help as a sounding board for the CEO and in ensuring board support for the CEO.

6. *Specifies annual objectives.* With assistance provided by the executive committee and the CEO, the chair develops annual objectives for the board, determining the board's priorities in relation to its own functioning. The chair will develop the board's work plan and formulate agendas for all board meetings.

7. *Serves as a mentor.* The chair serves as a role model and mentor for future chairs and other board members who watch the actions of the chair. Board members who may be interested in being the next chair watch closely, so it is important the chair be a good mentor. Working through others, the chair is responsible for recruitment, orientation, and development of all board members, including the evaluation of board members.

8. *Assumes other responsibilities and tasks as directed by the board.* The chair may perform other functions as requested by the board. But it is the chair's responsibility to ensure that the board stays focused on those things that fit the mission, vision, and goals of the organization and that it follows established policy and procedure to keep things on task. The chair must not lead the board off into an area of personal interest. If this is allowed to occur, then every time the chair changes, the organization could be heading in a different direction. The chair functions as an instrument of the board, not the other way around.

References

Biggs, E. L. 2002. "CEOs' Perceptions of Board Issues." Unpublished study. Denver, CO: University of Colorado.

Kaiser, L. 1983. Personal communication, February 16.

Kazemek, E. A. 2002. "Count to Ten: Board and CEO Frustrations." *Trustee* 55 (9): 26–27.

National Association of Corporate Directors. 2001. *2001–2002 NACD Public Company Governance Survey*. Washington, DC: National Association of Corporate Directors.

CHAPTER TWO

Responsibilities for Board-CEO Relationships

How Does the Board Relate to the Chief Executive Officer?

...or, How Does This Work?

Ideally, the board and the CEO will work together well and consistently for the benefit of the organization. The relationship can be a complex one, not always developed or maintained easily, but one that can be infinitely rewarding for all concerned, including the hospital.

The CEO as a board member

The CEO works both for and with the board. Pointer and Orlikoff (1999) have found that more than 80 percent of hospital CEOs are either voting members of their boards or ex officio members without vote. In comparison, almost 80 percent of healthcare system CEOs clearly serve as voting members of the board. A study of 90 acute care hospitals in California showed that CEO participation as a voting member of the board significantly enhances hospital performance (Molinari, Hendryx, and Goodstein 1997).

As Pointer and Orlikoff (1999) further point out, when the CEO sits on the board as a voting member, it emphasizes a key characteristic of the unique relationship between the two: the partnership, in addition to the employer-employee aspect, that results in better governance. Such a positive result leads to the recommendation that, whenever possible, it is in the best interest of the organization for the CEO to also be a voting member of the board.

In such a situation, the CEO knows the board position is an ex officio one, and when he or she leaves the position, it will be filled by the new CEO. And, of course, the smart CEO would never vote to break a tie among the rest of the board members.

The board is responsible for only one employee — the CEO

The CEO is the only individual who reports directly to the board and, therefore, is the only one the board evaluates. The board is not responsible for evaluating others in any way, although the temptation to do so very definitely exists for many board members. The list of those whom the board does not evaluate includes, among others, the chief financial officer, chief operating officer, chief nursing officer, and chief medical officer. Although this may be particularly difficult in a smaller community where the board knows so many of these employees, the board must remember that only the CEO is responsible for evaluating all the individuals reporting to him or her.

Similarly, if a board member perceives a problem with a hospital employee, that member should speak to the CEO about the problem rather than to the employee or the employee's immediate supervisor. Again, the temptation to do otherwise can be strong, but this undermines the authority of the CEO and will usually place both the CEO and the board member in an extremely awkward position.

CEO employment contract

The vast majority of CEOs have employment contracts. In today's turbulent healthcare environment, the decisions required of a CEO are frequently risky and may offend or displease some stakeholders; therefore, an employment contract is essential. The CEO has to be in a position to make decisions, whether they are popular or not, in the best interest of the organization. CEOs can make such decisions and take the necessary risks knowing they are protected by an employment contract. (A sample CEO employment contract from the American College of Healthcare Executives is shown in Appendix 4).

Evaluation of the CEO

The CEO should be evaluated annually by a committee of the board; this is usually the executive committee, unless the board has a compensation committee. At the beginning of each year the committee and the CEO should agree on a set of obtainable goals and objectives for the CEO. This is sometimes called a "management plan."

Once the management plan is agreed on, it serves as a roadmap for the CEO and an evaluation tool for the committee. If a crisis occurs, some members of the committee or board may want to deviate from using the management plan as the evaluation tool. How the CEO has handled a crisis may certainly be factored into an evaluation, but the management plan should be the primary tool utilized. It is the role of the board chair to keep the evaluation on track with the agreed-on factors in the management plan and to not allow the board to "change horses in midstream."

More recently, some hospitals have implemented performance appraisal programs that seek input from subordinates and others with whom the CEO works. This is known as 360-degree feedback, or as a multirater system, and is one of the most popular and well-known newer performance appraisal instruments. However, evaluating committees and boards must remember that subordinates may use the system only to complain about the CEO, particularly if the CEO has been firm about the subordinate doing or not doing something the employee doesn't like. The committee and board should have a plan in place for assessing such results, so they will not be put in the position of having to determine who to believe or in playing the he said, she said game. Because the use of such a tool is so open to subjective rather than objective results, it is recommended for use no more than every three years, in addition to the annual management plan for that year (Tyler and Biggs 2001). A sample multirater performance appraisal tool is provided in Appendix 5.

Should Boards Get Involved in Management Operations?

...or, That's My Job... No, That's Not My Job

Sometimes a fine line exists between what is management and what is governance. However, when board members get involved in day-to-day operations, it not only causes problems and requires time-consuming efforts for the CEO and other management personnel to deal with, it takes away from the directors' main role of governance. Board members often get involved in operations for the following reasons:

1. *No job descriptions.* The most important thing that can happen to a new board member is to be given a job description by the board chair, and not by the CEO. If a board member sees clearly what the job entails, as well as what it does not include, there is a good chance the board member will function according to the job description. The importance of board job descriptions has been discussed in Chapter 1, and sample job descriptions for the board chair and board members are found in Appendix 3. It may be that the entire board should be given job descriptions as part of a board education session, particularly if they have never been given such descriptions before.

2. *Specialized knowledge.* Board members may sometimes become involved in day-to-day operations because they have a specialized knowledge area and feel they must or should display that knowledge. For example, a certified public accountant on the board may feel a need to be involved in the detailed preparation of financial statements. A general contractor may feel he should be involved in all the hospital's construction projects. Board members are also usually most comfortable in their areas of expertise, so gravitation to corresponding areas in the hospital's domain may occur without specific intent on the member's part.

3. *Special interests.* Sometimes members for various reasons have special areas of interest or commitment within the hospital. Perhaps a member's spouse died of a coronary in the hospital, so anytime an issue arises relating to cardiology services, such as staffing, equipment, a new unit, renovation of the present unit, or cardiology credentialing, that board member wants to be involved.

4. *Difficulty delegating.* Some board members find it very difficult to delegate everything to management and/or the medical staff. They may be very hands on managers in their regular positions and find it difficult to function at the 30,000-foot level with the rest of the board. These are directors who also want to function in their comfort zone, participating rather than delegating, because of their own life experiences.

5. *A desire to manage during crisis.* Many board members want to manage during periods or perceived periods of turbulence and crisis. They believe getting involved in management activities is helping to save the organization. Some members may manage small businesses and are used to performing many functions, particularly during difficult times.

6. *To fill management voids.* Many times, boards try to fill perceived voids in management. If the hospital has not been able to satisfactorily fill a vice presidential or other important management position, some board members feel they should step in to help with that function.

7. *Did not receive adequate orientation.* If a good orientation program for new board members does not exist, or there was never one in place for present board members, each will function as they think board members should function, without necessarily understanding what is actually expected of them. If all of the board members have been through a complete and structured orientation, they can help each other to better understand and execute their proper roles.

8. *Governance information versus management information.* Sometimes CEOs give the board too much management information instead of governance information, setting up the expectation that they are being asked to manage. It can be difficult to make sure the board receives only governance information, particularly when some board members want more information and insist on additional reports at meetings. Because few board members will argue with a colleague that such reports are unnecessary, the problem is perpetuated.

The board chair should work with the CEO to focus on providing only governance information. The board's role is to determine where the organization should be headed strategically and should not be involved in operations, which is the CEO's job. Although the distinction between governance and management can be fuzzy, just being aware that fuzz exists can help keep the picture clear.

What Should the Board Expect When Working with a CEO?

...or, But Don't Expect Coffee

Boards need to remember they work in partnership with the organization's CEO, with the mutual goal of pursuing the very best decisions and actions for the current and future well-being of the organization. One board president had obviously forgotten that, as one day he arrived early for a meeting and demanded to know why the CEO hadn't made coffee for him. Needless to say, expecting the CEO to personally serve coffee to the board is way outside of appropriate expectations. Appropriate expectations do include the following:

1. *The CEO works both with and for the board.* As previously noted, most CEOs are members of their boards by virtue of their positions. In this capacity, the CEO works as a strategic partner with the board. However, the CEO is also an employee of the board, and in this role the board is definitely the employer. Boards do not like to review material and be asked to make major decisions that appear to have already been made. The CEO should involve the board early regarding major upcoming decisions so they can proceed together.

2. *The CEO implements the board's policies and directives.* It is the job of the CEO to put the plans and directions set by the board into action. In this role, the CEO functions at 5,000 feet to implement the board's 30,000-foot-level decisions. The CEO deals with hospital personnel, the medical staff, outside contractors, and many others as necessary to ensure the hospital runs smoothly on a daily basis, patients are cared for effectively and efficiently, and the hospital fulfills its mission as set by the board.

3. *The board's priorities are the CEO's priorities.* The CEO will provide information to the board about a variety of topics and projects and offer his or her perspective about the board's proposed course of action; however, once the decision has been made by the board, the CEO becomes the board's hands in getting the work done. The CEO should strive to not get too far ahead of the board or head in a different direction strategically, and he or she must stay attuned to what the board sees as the top or changing priorities of the organization.

4. *No surprises*. The CEO should make sure the board does not receive any surprises. The board should know both good and bad news before the general public does. It is very embarrassing if the media or someone outside the organization confronts a board member about something that has happened in the organization if the CEO has not yet gotten this information to the board.

5. *Involvement in strategic "thinking."* An important goal of any board is to ensure the organization is pursuing a winning strategy. The best way to achieve this goal is for the board to be constructively engaged in the organization's strategic planning process. If the board is not involved initially in developing a strategic direction, there will not be full support for implementing the plan. The board needs to work closely with the CEO to understand the needs of the organization to ensure the appropriate development, execution, and modification of the organization's strategy.

6. *User friendly board packets*. Before board or committee meetings, board members should not receive thick packets of materials that contain management material instead of governance material. Their packets should contain information related to the decisions they will be making and educational materials to keep them abreast of the changes in the healthcare industry. Any CEO who continually gives the board members (large) packets of management information instead of brief packets of governance information will lose the board's support or encourage them to manage rather than govern.

7. *Educational opportunities*. The CEO should ensure that the board receives relevant industry materials, journals, and educational sessions and attends a well-planned retreat every year. The strongest boards, assisted by their CEOs, will be the ones who know the most about the healthcare industry, what the key issues are, how to function as a board member, and where the organization should be headed strategically.

8. *A program to groom potential board members*. The CEO should work with the governance committee on methods to develop a pool of potential board members. Some hospitals select board members from the hospital's foundation board or allow individuals who are not board members to join board committees. Either way, the CEO should work with the governance committee to ensure several alternative ways to identify and groom potential board members.

9. *Board member recognition.* The CEO should feature board members in publicity about newsworthy events concerning the hospital, including local media as well as the organization's newsletters and publications. Board members often volunteer many hours each year to the hospital and this type of attention is an easy way to provide some recognition and thanks for their service.

10. *The use of healthcare jargon.* And finally, the board should expect the CEO to refrain from unnecessarily using healthcare jargon. There are numerous abbreviations and acronyms in the healthcare field (see Appendix 8), and members will become familiar with many of them. However, members should not sit through meetings without understanding what is being discussed if they don't want to admit they don't understand all the terms being used. The smart CEO will cut the use of the jargon as much as possible, and the smart board member will ask questions if something is not understood.

In striving to meet these expectations, the CEO will work with the entire board and not just a few of the more powerful or vocal members or only the members he or she gets along with best. Both the CEO and the board will benefit as different members emerge as leaders within the board.

It is important for the CEO and board members to develop a mutual understanding and respect for each other's knowledge and strengths. The CEO should frequently provide opportunities outside of structured meetings, such as breakfasts or luncheons, to get to know board members on a personal and more informal basis. The best relationships between healthcare boards and the CEOS with whom they work are based on mutual understanding and an appreciation of each other's unique roles.

What Should the Board Know About CEO Succession Planning?

...or, What Do We Do Next?

According to a 2001 survey of public corporation CEOs conducted by the National Association of Corporate Directors (2001), CEO succession has risen to the second spot as the most important issue facing their boards of directors. For whatever reason, this issue does not surface on the top-ten list of important topics for boards of hospitals and healthcare organizations to address. Perhaps there is concern that the organizations cannot afford to have a good management development program in place. Perhaps no one thought of developing internal candidates for when the time comes to replace the CEO. Perhaps no one wants to even think about having to replace the CEO.

Although the reasons themselves may warrant exploration at some point, there is no doubt any healthcare board that does not plan ahead for the day the CEO leaves is doing the organization a disservice and setting the board up for a difficult transition. One of the most important functions of a healthcare board is to ensure the continuation of the organization and to minimize disruption through succession planning.

One of the ways to avoid the hassle of searching for a new CEO is to have the successor already identified and groomed to take over when the CEO steps aside. In the ideal scenario, the old CEO steps aside; the new CEO takes the reins knowledgably, already "knowing the ropes"; and everything moves along smoothly with no break in the continuity of purpose or results. Unfortunately, since this ideal scenario very rarely is met, some planning must be done.

The board's role in succession planning breaks down into several tasks. First, the board should make certain the planning is actually being done, by bringing it to the attention of the CEO and adding it to the CEO'S annual performance appraisal objectives. Even the most reluctant CEO will begin planning if he or she knows a serious discussion will take place annually on the progress made toward this goal.

Second, the board should sign off on any designation of internal candidates or any succession planning efforts. Although the CEO is the main point person in the process, the board should understand it is a joint duty and not one delegated solely to the CEO. The board should adopt the succession plan as its plan, and not treat it as something the CEO created in a vacuum. The CEO should understand the board will make the ultimate decision on any successor to be named.

Succession planning is not necessarily easy, and boards sometimes face certain problems (including the following) when developing or working with a CEO succession plan:

1. *Assumptions change quickly.* Succession plans make assumptions, and in a fast-changing environment, assumptions change quickly. The organization that was a freestanding facility last month may decide this month to join a system or to create a system on its own. A main internal candidate may thus need to be passed over as CEO-designate as part of a bargaining position or in deference to perceived equity with the other entity. When the succession plan was first designed, no one anticipated the possibilities of the combination that rendered the plan inoperative.

2. *Boards change.* A change in board membership or board chair may mean a change in how a succession plan will be implemented. A new board chair or new board members may look at any internal candidates differently or be unwilling to be held to the plan of the previous board or board chair. This is one reason that promises made must be carefully thought through. Although many times promises of this nature tend not to be in writing, boards should attempt to avoid making or breaking promises.

3. *The internal candidate is unable to assume the position.* The heir apparent may not be ready or able to succeed the CEO. This can come about through failure on the successor's part or because designating a formal replacement may be the equivalent of placing a target on that person's back. In this latter situation, issues dealing with the departing CEO may be transferred to the head of the heir apparent, who then becomes the target for ill will actually directed at the departing or departed CEO. This may create an untenable situation for both the board and the successor, causing the organization a great disservice.

4. *Designating an heir apparent may cause the departure of others in the organization who might be well qualified by the time the CEO steps aside.* Because of this, some organizations might indicate to several potential candidates they are being considered as CEO replacements. The question then becomes whether the replacements can continue to act as team members supportive of each other in an environment where only one will eventually be selected.

Third, once the succession planning process is completed, the board should make sure that any promises it has made are communicated to succeeding board leadership and that those promises are kept. In general, however, the board should limit itself to as few promises as possible to leave succeeding boards with the flexibility required in these rapidly changing times.

Fourth, if the board has tried succession planning but has had little success in creating a satisfactory plan, or needs a new CEO before a plan has been completed, a few alternatives are available to provide time until a new CEO can be named. Many healthcare organizations have found it is beneficial to go outside the organization to look for the new CEO. This may be because internal candidates are not deemed adequate, a change in direction or philosophy is called for, or no one internal wants the job. Sometimes an outside search is conducted even when an excellent candidate exists internally; this is usually done when the board wants to make sure the new CEO is the very best available at the time. The outside search may or may not validate the selection of the internal candidate.

To minimize the disruption created when a CEO departs unexpectedly, an internal individual can be designated as the acting CEO. Typically, the acting CEO is the leading candidate for the job. Sometimes, however, the board decides to bring in an interim leader whose sole job is to hold things together until a new CEO is appointed. With someone in the CEO's chair, decisions can be made that allow the organization to continue moving forward while the search goes on.

CEO succession planning is definitely one of the most important functions a board must address. The board should openly talk about a CEO succession plan and consider some of the following questions:

- What can the board do to ensure a smooth succession?
- How should the management development and succession process be handled?
- How should the board work with the present CEO during the succession process?
- What makes for a strong CEO candidate?
- What role should executive search firms play?
- When should outside candidates be considered?
- How much competition should be encouraged among potential CEO candidates?
- Should the former CEO play any role after he or she is succeeded?

If the board openly addresses the need for a succession plan that asks these questions, it is well on its way to developing an effective CEO-succession process.

References

Molinari, C., M. Hendryx, and J. Goodstein. 1997. "The Effects of CEO-Board Relations on Hospital Performance." *Health Care Management Review* 22(3): 7–15.

National Association of Corporate Directors. 2001. *2001-2002 NACD Public Company Governance Survey*. Washington, DC: National Association of Corporate Directors.

Pointer, D. D., and J. E. Orlikoff. 1999. *Board Work: Governing Health Care Organizations*. San Francisco: Jossey-Bass.

Tyler, J. L., and E. L. Biggs. 2001. *Practical Governance*. Chicago: Health Administration Press.

CHAPTER THREE

Responsibility for Quality Care

What is the Board's Role in Monitoring Quality of Healthcare?

... or, How Are We Doing?

Those who have been to many hospital governance education sessions might have heard about the three-legged stool. For many years, boards of hospitals operated under the idea that they were responsible for community interests (usually translated as fundraising and community support); the medical staff was responsible for quality and care; and administration was responsible for operating the facilities. This is described as a three-legged stool, one that only stands balanced when responsibility is equally distributed.

How does the board begin to think about quality of care?

While some aspects of the three-legged stool model are still valid, communities are now holding governing boards responsible for the overall organizational performance of their hospitals, just as boards of for-profit companies are responsible to their stockholders. A governing board's responsibility for quality of care is now of equal importance to its fiduciary responsibility for the financial integrity and well-being of the organization. Boards may delegate operational responsibility for quality to the medical staff, the nursing department, and administration, just as they delegate fiscal operations to others, but they may not delegate their accountability to the community for the overall performance of the organization.

The concept of quality and board responsibility must start with a discussion of hospital performance. The dimensions of performance in healthcare are much broader than just financial performance. Hospital performance includes dimensions of patient safety, clinical effectiveness, appropriateness, timeliness, and satisfaction. And these dimensions are no longer the sole purview of the medical staff but must involve other departments within the hospital as well, particularly those with direct patient contact on a 24/7 basis.

Think about it. How good is a hospital that manages an AAA bond rating and produces 4 percent operating margins year in and year out but has a mortality rate three times the expected national average? How good is a hospital where 10 percent of all its patients experience a medication error or 20 percent of its patients rate the care poor or unacceptable? How good is a hospital when more than 50 percent of all its heart attack patients do not receive elements of care proven to be effective or when its patients wait for hours in the emergency room because of bottlenecks in bed placement caused by poor utilization of resources? Outlandish examples? Unfortunately, no. Many hospital boards blissfully govern, looking at the bottom line without any knowledge that the care and service provided by their hospitals is mediocre or, in some cases, poor and unsafe.

Talking about a hospital's performance goes beyond the credentialing and peer review functions that are delegated to the medical staff and approved by the board, but some board members can be at a loss about what questions to ask and what information to expect. Historically, hospitals worked on the theory that if you had good physicians, then you would have good care. For decades, boards focused on developing governing processes and committees to carry out their responsibility for identifying poorly performing physicians during the credentialing process and for reviewing physician care through peer review. While these are important functions, eliminating "bad apples" does not necessarily make the rest of the batch excellent. Similarly, focusing solely on physician practice while ignoring those aspects of hospital care provided by other members of the healthcare team does not present a total picture of how the organization is actually performing.

Healthcare is a team sport, and the dimensions of safety, clinical effectiveness, and clinical appropriateness are dependent on the entire system of care, not just physician care. For governing boards to be accountable to the communities they serve for overall performance, they must begin to look at measures that reflect organizational performance and not just physician performance.

What are the important dimensions of performance a governing board should be aware of and use to define organizational performance?

Unlike the common language and tools used by governing boards to discuss financial performance, the common language for evaluating performance is still evolving. In the Institute of Medicine (IOM 2001) report, *Crossing the Quality Chasm*, six important aims of patient care were identified that require redesign and improvement:

* *Safety* of patients and staff
* *Effectiveness* of care
* *Efficiency* of processes and cost
* *Patient-centeredness* as a focus of the care system
* *Timeliness* of treatment
* *Equity* in access and care delivered across populations

These aims as defined by IOM are a useful place for boards to begin thinking about organizational performance. Expanding on this framework, there are other important dimensions and useful ways to consider performance, including patient satisfaction, financial performance, employee satisfaction, flow (wait times), and community health. Adding these dimensions to the IOM's important aims provides a multidimensional method for defining hospital performance. Figure 3.1 lists these critical dimensions.

Figure 3.1: Critical Dimensions of Organizational Performance

- Patient and customer (satisfaction)
- Effectiveness (clinical outcomes)
- Appropriateness (evidence and process)
- Safety (patient and staff)
- Equity
- Employee and staff satisfaction (culture)
- Efficiency (cost)
- Financial
- Flow (wait times, cycle times, and throughput)
- Community/population health

It is important for boards to broaden their definition of hospital performance and to be able to answer the question, "How is the hospital doing?" with an answer more detailed than, "Great, we are making money this year!" or "Great, we just opened a new wing!" Instead, board members should, based on date, be able to answer with confidence: "Great, our finances are in order, our patient and employee satisfaction are very high, wait times in the ER are dramatically improved from three years ago, and our clinical outcomes compared to our peer hospitals are in the 90th percentile." That would be a far better answer.

What should boards be thinking with respect to patient satisfaction?

Most hospital boards understand patient satisfaction as an important dimension of organizational performance, and many hospitals collect some form of patient satisfaction information and routinely share it with the board, especially if it is good. Several national survey companies provide comparative information. The Centers for Medicare and Medicaid Services (CMS) has announced a plan to require hospitals to utilize a uniform set of patient survey questions for all Medicare patients (and likely, by default, all other patients) and a plan to make the results of the survey available to the public for comparative purposes. Hospitals in Massachusetts and California, as well as several other metropolitan hospital markets, have experimented with the voluntary reporting of patient survey results.

Many boards now incorporate patient satisfaction results into the performance evaluation of the CEO. This is a good governance practice. However, boards should always look at the raw or total scores on patient satisfaction surveys, not just comparative percentiles. It is quite possible on some survey instruments to interpret a false confidence; on a comparative basis, the hospital might be above average, yet it might still have significant numbers of patients dissatisfied with care and service.

Boards should also be aware that debate and evolution continue in the types of questions that are really important to patient care. Traditional questions about food service, wait times, noise, friendliness, and facilities (all important to service quality) are giving way to questions that attempt to capture the patient's experience with the actual clinical care delivered. These questions begin to probe the patient's experience with pain control, inclusion of family in decision making, completeness of communications, alleviation of fear, and desired degree of control by patients in care planning and administration of care. All of these are consistent with the value of patient-centeredness redesign criteria suggested by the IOM.

Although the use of patient survey tools is widespread in hospitals, these tools are not necessarily well used by boards and administrations. In some cases, surveys are only conducted annually, data are not trended over time, survey tools are inadequate for asking about the patient experience versus service levels, results are ignored or assumed to be good enough, or there is no link between the strategy of the organization and the customer satisfaction results generated. Governing boards can begin to change these dynamics by the questions they ask. Governance questions that hospital boards might ask with respect to patient satisfaction include the following:

1. What level of patient satisfaction does our hospital want to achieve? How big is the gap between our current performance and desired performance? How long do we think it will take to close that gap?
2. How does our current survey tool and process capture the patient experience with respect to the clinical care delivered? We seem to be good at measuring service levels, what kinds of questions should we be asking patients about clinical care?
3. How is the improvement of the patient experience reflected in our strategic plan?

4. How are the administration, medical staff, nursing department, and others using the information from the patient survey process to prioritize and focus improvement efforts that will lead to better scores? What resources have been devoted to these projects? When will we see the results of these efforts?

5. Beyond the use of a formal patient satisfaction survey tool, what other methods does the hospital use to capture patient satisfaction and patient experience information, and what are the results of those efforts?

What questions should boards ask about clinical effectiveness and patient care outcomes?

Exercising governance responsibility and oversight of clinical issues to ensure effective care is a daunting new challenge for many hospital boards. Just as patient satisfaction can be measured, the other important dimensions of clinical organizational performance can be measured and monitored over time.

Discussing clinical outcomes traditionally has been challenging for boards for a variety of reasons. First, boards have historically worked under the assumption that the medical staff credentialing and peer review process took care of the problem of poor care. While protecting patients from poor physicians, most quality assurance has failed to improve reliability and care for all patients. Looking at clinical outcomes at an organizational level requires a different type of discussion and a look at different types of indicators.

Second, the organizational structure of most community hospitals and their voluntary medical staffs has created interesting dynamics that have been a barrier to frank discussions about quality and performance. In the case of physicians, for example, most in the United States do not work for the hospital in which they practice, and they are affiliated by choice with the hospital through the formal hospital medical staff structure. In communities where there are multiple hospitals, physicians may be affiliated with more than one and have significant control over where they admit or refer patients for care. Hampered by a belief system that clinical quality is about the physician, many boards and administrations have been very reluctant to engage in frank discussions about clinical quality for fear of alienating key admitting or referring physicians. And, some physicians have been quick to threaten use of the "move my patients" card when they misperceive organizational clinical improvement efforts as an attack on their individual clinical autonomy.

Another dynamic that has entered into this mix in recent years is the quality of nursing care available. A physician's willingness to affiliate with a given hospital has been found to be significantly affected by the nurse staff level and the quality of nursing care provided there. Recent studies have further documented the effect of an appropriate nurse staffing mix—the ratio of RNs to LPNs and unlicensed aides—has on the clinical effectiveness of the patient care provided and the patients' satisfaction with that care. The Magnet Recognition Program developed by the American Nurses Credentialing Center in 1994 is designed to recognize healthcare organizations that provide the very best in nursing care, utilizing nursing quality indicators and standards of nursing practice. According to the Joint Commission on Accreditation of Healthcare Organizations (JCAHO 2003), "...the Magnet Recognition Program provides consumers with the ultimate benchmark to measure the quality of care they can expect to receive."

Perhaps one of the biggest barriers to a discussion of clinical effectiveness is that, unlike finance, there is no common language or agreement on the sets of clinical measures that every hospital should use. This is changing with the efforts of JCAHO and its required ORYX measurement set[1], pressure from business groups such as Leapfrog (see discussion later in this chapter), and pressure from CMS for public reporting of a common clinical outcome measurement set. In response to these pressures, in late 2002 the American Hospital Association, in partnership with several physician organizations, announced an effort to voluntarily develop and publicly report a set of clinical measures. However, at this point the development of a common set of clinical measures, the understanding of what "good" performance looks like, and general agreement on the validity of these clinical measures is still evolving.

Further, complexity is an issue. If hospitals only took care of one type of patient (as do some new specialty hospitals such as heart hospitals), it would be relatively easy to point to one or two clinical measures to reflect the clinical outcomes of care rendered. For a heart hospital, it might be a comparison of the actual open heart mortality rate compared to the risk adjusted expected mortality rate. But most hospital boards have to deal with the complexity of multiple reasons for admission and multiple types of care. It is no easy task to decide what clinical measures to report and monitor.

Although the task is complex and hindered by the lack of a common set of fully accepted clinical measures, the hospital board still has a responsibility to ask questions and to set up structures and processes to monitor the organization's clinical performance. Measures exist today that provide useful proxies for clinical performance standards.

Perhaps the one common measure that all hospital boards should monitor is in-hospital mortality. This measure is only useful if it is risk adjusted so that comparisons can be made either to an expected value or to other organizations using the same risk-adjusting system. Risk adjusting means a probability of death value is assigned to each patient case, based on factors such as age, sex, reason for admission, and other diseases or conditions present and then compared to a database of mortality rates for patients with similar characteristics. It is not a perfect science, but it does begin to create the opportunity to compare performance. A number of commercial risk-adjusting software applications allow a hospital to do its own analysis, and there are commercial vendors who will perform the calculations based on an abstract of patient information. There are also a number of commercial databases and programs from which hospitals can purchase comparative information.

Raw mortality data without risk adjustment is useful only to monitor trends and identify a sudden increase that might be indicative of problems. There was a famous case a number of years ago in a small hospital in Indiana where the mortality rate spiked because of an "angel of death" working in the hospital. If the hospital had been trending mortality data over time, the board might have noticed a spike in the death rate earlier, which could then have been investigated and stopped sooner. However, for the most part, raw mortality rates are of little use to hospital boards and of absolutely no value if not trended over time.

As with all performance data, mortality data should be graphed and trended over time. Comparative information is not a luxury but is basic information that all hospital boards must have to fulfill their governance responsibility for quality and performance. The Institute for Healthcare Improvement (IHI) in Boston has begun making a new risk-adjusted measure of mortality available to hospitals. It is called the Hospital Specific Mortality Rate (HSMR)[2] and allows a hospital to see its specific morality rate for the last year of Medicare data reported, compared to a common index for all hospitals. The IHI work highlights remarkable degrees of unexplained variation in hospital mortality rates across the country.

In addition, Medicare already makes mortality data available, and several commercial vendors have used mortality data to rate specific programs, such as cardiology or pneumonia care, and publish this information on various web sites for public access. If your hospital performs open heart surgery, the hospital board should routinely see a comparison of in-hospital and 30-day mortality for heart surgery patients, compared to the expected rate and regional/national rates. (This information, based on commercial use of the Medicare database, is public and available on the Internet.[3]) Hospital boards should ask to see a list and examples of the performance information about their hospital that is routinely available to the public on the Internet or through other sources.

Another way hospital boards can begin to monitor clinical outcomes is to look at comparative data for certain groups of high-volume admissions and/or procedures. Most community hospitals find as many as 75 percent of all admissions are for obstetrics, cardiology, pneumonia, and total joint replacement. For the high-volume reasons for admission, a small set of performance measures can be developed for each clinical grouping. These measures might include general indicators such as average length of stay, percentage of patients that were treated by a defined set of evidence-based criteria, and the rate of readmission within 30 days for the same diagnosis.

In addition to these general measures for the clinical groups, specific clinical indicators, such as surgical infection rates for joint procedures, C-section rates for obstetrics, or timeliness of antibiotic administration for pneumonia patients, might be added. In each case, it is important that a comparative reference be developed so that boards and medical staffs have some means to judge performance and note significant change.

One of the biggest clinical issues facing hospitals is the consistent use of evidence-based care. It is generally acknowledged that something less than 50 percent of all care delivered in American hospitals is evidence based, meaning we know the science behind why it works and the results are predictable. That does not mean all other care is wrong, we just do not always have the science or cannot reasonably predict that a given treatment will improve the outcome for the patient.

The IOM report mentioned earlier also identified three major areas of problems in the healthcare system: overuse, underuse, and misuse. As a result of this and other similar reports, hospitals are faced with the challenge of beginning to think about clinical performance in terms of scientific evidence. One question governing boards can begin to ask is, "What percentage of our patients are receiving evidence-based care?" This is a daunting question for most medical staffs and administrations because of the complexity of the multiple types of patients admitted, uncertainty of the evidence, and lack of information systems that can easily produce the information.

However, one approach a hospital might use is to adopt a system that measures the percentage of patients who receive care per defined evidence-based protocols. Most hospitals have begun adopting evidence-based protocols for patients admitted for heart attacks and pneumonia care. This is because of the external review, in the late 1990s, by CMS of care for Medicare patients and because these protocols track with the new JCAHO ORYX measurement system. It is relatively simple for hospitals to track whether eligible patients were treated according to the evidence-based protocols and to report out the percentage of patients who received all elements of the required care. In small hospitals, all patients can be counted. In larger hospitals, sampling methodology can be used to develop the percentages. As the hospital adopts additional evidence-based protocols, the metric can be expanded.

The counter-balancing metric is to look at the percentage of admissions (or discharges) where care is available by evidence-based protocols, compared to all admissions. At the outset, this percentage is likely to be low for most hospitals, but as evidence-based medicine becomes more fully used across hospitals, the percentages should rise. From a governance perspective, the board should be interested in knowing how the hospital is working to ensure all patients receive evidence-based care. Monitoring performance by looking at the percentage of care in the hospital currently defined by evidence and comparing the percentage of patients who received 100 percent of the evidence is one way of providing oversight.

Discussions to this point have been about finding measures that reflect the technical quality of the care delivered compared to standards, norms, or other organizations. Now, however, a new thought is emerging in healthcare—clinical outcomes should also be measured by the patients' perceptions of whether or not they are better as a result of the intervention. Known as functional outcomes, a number of organizations have begun experimenting with versions of questions originally developed by the Rand Corporation (SF-36). Shorter versions of the questions are being experimented with in an effort to create care that is more patient centered. Clearly, this is not an approach that can be used for all patients, but the concept might be helpful in evaluating the performance of the healthcare system, from a patient's perspective, in the treatment of some chronic diseases. It may also be useful in assessing the performance of some major surgical interventions such as heart surgery and total joint replacement. Governing boards should begin asking questions that lead to organizations, including functional outcomes in their measures of organizational and clinical performance.

Boards can and should ask many questions about clinical performance. However, the trick is to ask questions that do not require an in-depth understanding of the technical nature of the clinical care or indicator, but that lead the board to have confidence that the medical staff, nursing department, and administration are monitoring and taking action to improve clinical care in the hospital. Below are questions boards might find useful as they review the clinical performance of the hospital:

1. Why is this clinical indicator important?
2. What is "good" performance for this clinical indicator? What is our target for our performance? What are we doing to improve our performance?
3. What external source are we comparing our performance to? What is the best or benchmark performance for this indicator?
4. What percentage of our patients are treated with evidence-based protocols or care plans? What percentage of those patients get 100 percent of the care indicated?
5. What is our risk-adjusted hospital mortality rate? How does it compare to external data?

6. What are our ORYX measures, and how is our performance going to be reported to JCAHO?
7. What clinical data are available on the Internet, or through other public sources, on the performance of our hospital?
8. What are our priorities for improving the clinical care patients receive? How do these priorities link to our organizational strategy? How do those improvement projects link to the clinical measures of performance that are being presented to the board? Have we considered applying for Magnet Hospital status?

What should boards be doing to improve patient safety?

Governing boards of hospitals need to ask questions about patient safety and performance. The IOM's report, *To Err Is Human*, created a huge political firestorm for hospitals when it stated that between 48,000 and 98,000 preventable deaths occur each year in our hospitals, with most avoidable deaths due to medication error (IOM 2000). That range of death rates would make hospital care the eighth leading cause of death in the United States, ahead of AIDS and just behind motor vehicle accidents. Since the issuance of the report, there have been numerous articles suggesting the methodology was flawed and the death rate is closer to or below the bottom end of the IOM estimate. In any case, the performance for hospitals does not come close to our public expectations for safety in airline travel and other forms of public transportation, and hospital boards need to pay attention to patient safety issues.

Most hospitals have begun major pushes to improve patient medication safety and to prevent other untoward events that lead to patient harm such as falls, wrong-site surgery, infections, and misuse of medical care. Chronic underreporting of errors (arising from a culture of blame and fostered by traditional quality assurance and peer review systems that seek to assign individual responsibility for untoward events) has been a major barrier to improvements in patient safety. A multitude of resources are available to hospitals to help identify and deal with high-risk situations and identify best safety practices. Therefore, no hospital should be trying to reinvent the wheel or rely solely on internal resources and knowledge to assess safety issues and improve systems.

Patient safety is a big issue, and governing boards should monitor the performance of the patient safety system in their hospitals. Patient safety metrics might include the number of adverse drug events per 1,000 doses, patient falls per 1,000 patient days, surgical site infection rates per 1,000 surgeries, and other reported events per 1,000 patient days. Because underreporting is a major issue in patient safety efforts, the board must be careful to send the correct message about the importance of reporting all incidents to the organization in the monitoring of patient safety indicators.

Reporting must be totally nonpunitive, and it must be stressed that the purpose of the increased numbers reported is to analyze system weakness and design and implement corresponding actions to improve the system. Creating a culture of safety for the patient should always be the goal. Boards should expect the reported rates to dramatically increase during an initial push to improve medication systems and the other dimensions of patient safety. Once specific improvements are made, the board should see rates decrease as a direct result of actions taken. If rates simply decrease on their own over time, it is likely old habits of underreporting have reoccurred and performance is likely worse than being reported. Boards should ask the following questions:

1. What measures is the hospital using to track patient safety?
2. What actions are being taken to create a culture of safety and increase the reporting of error and mishaps?
3. How do our patient safety efforts link to the organizational strategic plan and improvement priorities?
4. What actions and efforts will be launched over the next 90 days to improve our medication system or improve patient safety?
5. What are our priorities for improving our medication safety?
6. What external sources of information and best practices are we using to guide our improvement efforts?

What are some of the tools and structures that boards can use to monitor organizational performance?

Boards generally look at financial reports on either a monthly or quarterly basis. Boards should also look at information representing the other important dimensions of hospital performance on this same schedule. As discussed earlier, measurements of safety, satisfaction, clinical outcomes, and clinical care processes can be developed. These can then be tracked by the board and used by the organization to evaluate overall organizational performance. In the mid-1990s, two Harvard business professors, Kaplan and Norton (1996) studied high-performing companies and made the observation that the leaders of these companies focused on multiple measures of performance beyond just financial figures. These organizations took a "balanced" view of their operations, and Kaplan and Norton coined the term "balanced scorecard" to reflect a set of important measures senior leaders use to lead and manage a company. This approach could certainly be applicable to hospitals.

Every hospital should have a clear understanding of the important dimensions of performance for its organization and metrics developed that represent these dimensions. Balanced scorecards are good tools for displaying the critical measures that have been identified for each dimension. However, like a financial statement, the balanced scorecard is simply a tool to aid the board in carrying out its responsibility. And just like financial reporting, one number does not tell the whole story. For each dimension deemed important by the board, there may be three or four measures that together define performance within that dimension.

The board should work with the administration, medical staff, nursing department, and appropriate others to develop the high-level measures that populate the scorecard and define organizational performance. On at least a quarterly basis, the key measures should be reviewed by the board as a whole with the same intensity and thought with which financial measures are reviewed. Organizational strategy should also be aligned with the board scorecard, and strategic progress should be reflected by improvement in key performance indicators.

Monitoring organizational performance with measures that cross multiple dimensions is a big job. The quality and community health committee previously discussed (see Chapter 1) is useful for reviewing the results of this work in detail. This board committee also works with the hospital leadership to set improvement priorities and report on activity in summary fashion to the whole board. This committee functions in the same manner and with the same authority as the finance or budget committee of the board. Other hospital boards find it more effective to include board members as voting members of a single organizationwide quality and community health committee that directs all performance improvement activities. Either approach will work as long as the board members exercise their autonomy and ask relevant governance questions that help the leadership of the organization identify the priorities and consider the importance of high performance across multiple dimensions. Important governance questions on structure include the following:

1. How as a board should we best organize ourselves to review the broader dimensions of performance?
2. Do we as a board spend as much time critically thinking about patient satisfaction, safety, and clinical performance as we do about financial issues?
3. How does our organizational strategy align with the metrics and dimensions of organizational performance that we have chosen?
4. Are the measures on our balanced scorecard meaningful measures of performance or simply measures that are available and convenient to monitor?

The quality and community health committee is the best place to begin or continue the journey of monitoring the quality of healthcare.

What Should the Board Know About the Joint Commission on Accreditation of Healthcare Organizations?

...or, Why is the JCAHO Important?

Established more than 50 years ago, the Joint Commission on Accreditation of Healthcare Organizations (JCAHO) has historically been the nation's leading evaluator of healthcare quality and safety. Eight out of ten hospitals nationwide are voluntarily accredited by JCAHO.

JCAHO is an independent, nonprofit organization that sets the standards by which healthcare quality is measured in the United States and around the world. It is governed by a board that includes physicians, nurses, and consumers. JCAHO evaluates the quality and safety of care for nearly 17,000 healthcare organizations. These include hospitals, nursing homes, home health agencies, behavioral healthcare organizations, outpatient clinics, laboratories, office-based surgery, assisted living, critical access hospitals, and managed care organizations such as HMOs and PPOs.

To maintain and earn accreditation, organizations must have an extensive on-site review by a team of JCAHO healthcare professionals at least once every three years. The purpose of the review is to evaluate the organization's performance in areas that affect patient care. Accreditation may then be awarded based on how well the organizations met JCAHO standards.

These standards for hospitals cover important areas such as medication use, infection control, patient safety, care of patients, staff qualifications, patient rights, and safe care environment. JCAHO has announced plans to make significant changes to the accreditation process, progressively sharpening the focus of the process on the operational systems most critical to the safety and quality of patient care. Critical elements of the Shared Visions–New Pathways initiative include a major consolidation of JCAHO standards, the introduction of a periodic performance review process, use of data from multiple sources to help guide the on-site accreditation survey, and conducting the on-site evaluation in the context of tracking actual individual patient care experiences.

Although the JCAHO accreditation process is complex, many factors encourage healthcare facilities to seek this status:

1. *Improvement of care to individuals or documentation that safe, quality care is being provided.* JCAHO standards are focused on one goal: raising, to the highest possible level, the safety and quality of care received by the public. JCAHO standards include state-of-the-art performance improvement concepts to help organizations continuously improve their quality and safety of care.

2. *Strengthening of community confidence.* Accreditation highlights a hospital's dedication to providing safe and high-quality care to the community it serves. Achieving accreditation makes a strong statement to the community about a hospital's commitment to provide the highest quality services.

3. *Provision of professional guidance for the operation of the organization being surveyed.* The survey process is designed to be educational and supportive. JCAHO surveyors are experienced healthcare professionals

trained to provide expert observations and assistance during the survey. Recommendations for change are provided.

4. *Ongoing support*. JCAHO offers many educational seminars and publications about performance improvement and other standards-related topics. In addition, staff from each accreditation program and from the Standards Interpretation Group can provide immediate assistance and suggestions on the survey process and on standards compliance.

5. *Possible substitution for Medicare and Medicaid certification*. Accreditation can help lessen the burdens imposed by duplicative federal and state regulatory agency surveys. Some accredited healthcare organizations may qualify for Medicare and Medicaid certification without undergoing a separate government survey.

6. *Fulfillment of licensure requirements in several states*. Several states recognize JCAHO accreditation as fulfilling some or all state hospital licensing requirements.

7. *Recognition by insurers and other third-party payers*. Increasingly, accreditation is becoming a prerequisite to eligibility for insurance reimbursement, for participation in managed care plans, and for bidding on contracts.

8. *Possible improvement of liability insurance coverage*. By enhancing risk-management efforts, accreditation may improve access to and reduce the cost of liability insurance coverage.

9. *Attraction of professionals and professional referrals*. Case managers and other healthcare professionals frequently use accreditation as a benchmark of quality when placing individuals. Those who staff the hospital, including physicians and nurses, may also consider the JCAHO status of the facility before deciding to affiliate with the organization.

10. *An increase in financing capabilities*. Lenders may require accreditation as a condition of financing, assuming accredited organizations may be more capable of paying debt than unaccredited ones.

Although all ten of these factors will not apply to every organization, their merit should be considered by hospital management and the board of directors when determining whether to seek JCAHO accreditation. It is certainly one way in which a hospital can actively demonstrate its commitment to quality patient care to itself, to its employees, and to its community.

What Should the Board Know About Business Coalitions on Health?

... or, Do We Care About Business Coalitions?

Over 80 locations in the United States have a business coalition on health. The common thread of these business coalitions is the desire to improve value and quality in healthcare for the benefit of their members and the larger community. In other words, they have been formed to decrease healthcare costs for their member companies and to increase healthcare quality for the employees of their member companies. Almost 99 percent of the member organizations of a business coalition on health are for-profit firms.

However, the great majority of the coalitions themselves are 501(c)(3) or 501(c)(6) not-for-profit entities; about 10 percent are for profit. Most local business coalitions are members of the National Business Coalition on Health; its 7,000 employer members boast a collective population of 10.3 million employees and 34 million covered lives throughout the country.

At least three coalitions number over 1 million employees each: the Massachusetts Healthcare Purchaser Group, the Pacific Business Group on Health, and the Washington Business Group on Health. Many business coalitions thrive in mid-sized markets of about 500,000 people, where coalitions can effectively forge relationships with larger employers and interact with a less complex medical marketplace. Some examples include The Alliance of Madison, Wisconsin, and Nevada Health Care Coalition of Reno, Nevada (see Figure 3.2).

Business coalition goals

Wisely purchasing healthcare benefits for an employee population is a difficult task. Most business coalitions are formed when a small number of dedicated employers rally around the concept of value-based purchasing. Value-based purchasing is different from typical healthcare purchasing: both cost and quality are incorporated into the assessment, selection, and ongoing

Figure 3.2: Profile of Business Coalitions

Number of members within the coalition:

< 50 companies	50%
> 50 and <100 companies	30%
>100 companies	20%

Membership composed of:

Private employers	75%
Public employers	14%
Providers, insurers, labor groups	6%
Other (consultants, foundations, nonprofits)	5%

Annual operating budgets:

<$ 100,000	35–40%
>$ 100,000 to $300,000	30–35%
>$ 300,000 to $1,000,000	<20%
>$1,000,000	<20%

Sources of funds:

Dues	50%
Grants, awards, conferences, and publications	30%
Access fees and purchasing programs	20%

Source: National Business Coalition on Health. 2000. "NBCH Member Profile." [Online information; retrieved 6/26/03.] http://www.nbch.org/members.htm.

monitoring of healthcare services. Key features of coalitions' activities include the following:

- value-based purchasing,
- acquisition of healthcare utilization and cost data,
- standardization of performance measures,
- creation of health plan and hospital performance reports,
- education of coalition members and the greater community,
- education of employees and other citizens, and
- legislative advocacy and monitoring.

Purchasers join together as they realize the benefits of using a coalition to implement value-based purchasing. They use their combined strengths to create negotiating leverage in the marketplace. They share information and resources to create standardized requests for proposals, performance standards, and healthcare data collecting and reporting.

One aspect of value-based purchasing translates into group purchasing arrangements for the majority of coalitions. Coalition members may join to purchase health plans, preferred provider networks, pharmacy benefit management services, or other healthcare services such as dental and vision plans. Other coalitions have built local or regional preferred provider networks, and their member companies enjoy coalition-negotiated discounts. Even when a coalition is not purchasing, a group still influences its healthcare marketplace.

Some business coalitions have even designed new systems for the financing and delivery of healthcare in their markets. The Buyers Healthcare Action Group of Minneapolis, Minnesota, designed a program they call Patient Choice. It integrates features for fair reimbursement schedules, incentives for high quality of care, and employee choice of provider.

Business coalition perspective and recent studies

Mission statements of nearly all business coalitions address quality of healthcare. Coalition members acknowledge the many opportunities and obligations members have to improve the structure, financing, and accountability of the healthcare marketplace.

In today's increasingly competitive marketplace, healthcare purchasers are beginning to look beyond the direct cost of premiums or self-insurance, to look instead at the cost in productivity and absenteeism in the worksite. Academic studies over the past 30 years document variations in healthcare spending and utilization which, for unexplained reasons, may not have directly related to better outcomes for patients: numbers of physician and specialist visits, numbers and frequency of tests, average length of stay in hospitals, and morbidity and mortality rates for common inpatient procedures. At the same time, common cost-effective and medically endorsed interventions (such as flu shots for seniors, peak flow meters for asthmatics, and cholesterol testing for cardiac patients) are not always routinely performed.

A widely cited study, published in 2001 by the Juran Institute and the Midwest Business Group on Health, asserts that the cost of poor quality amounts to about 30 percent of healthcare expenditures. This study uses the paradigm of "overuse, underuse, and misuse" to document activities that do not improve the value equation in healthcare. The next step is to determine how employers can define and differentiate high-quality healthcare when they decide how to spend their healthcare dollars. Employers do not want to pay for mediocre or poor-quality care. The Midwest Business Group on Health (2001) report is a road map for changing purchasing behavior.

To Err Is Human (IOM 2000) asserts patient safety is one of the most important issues confronting the healthcare system. Its estimate that between 48,000 and 98,000 people die in hospitals each year due to errors presents a toll in both human and financial terms that is indefensible. The focus now is to reform the current system in three fundamental ways:

1. engendering a culture of safety, instead of the current blame-and-shame paradigm,
2. acknowledging that most errors are "system errors" because common processes have not been engineered to ensure safety, and
3. confronting the appalling lack of information on infrastructure in hospitals and use these tools to improve and standardize care processes.

An outgrowth of the report was the creation of the Leapfrog Group, initiated in 2000 by a group of *Fortune* 100 companies to demand higher levels of performance accountability by hospitals and ultimately change payment systems to reward higher quality. Business leaders from The Business Roundtable called together academic and medical experts to advocate for a small number of improvements, called the "three leaps," to dramatically improve safety in the nation's hospitals. The three leaps were also selected because their adoption enhances structural changes within the industry.

Leap one is to implement a computerized physician pharmacy order entry system for all inpatient medication ordering. Leap two is to use specially trained hospitalists (intensivists) to staff intensive care units. Leap three is to bring focus for consumers and purchasers to select institutions that meet certain volume criteria for five types of surgical procedures and for care in a neonatal intenseive care unit.

From its founding in November 2000, the Leapfrog Group has grown to include 140 public and private organizations, which represent over 34 million healthcare consumers; has over 22 rollout sites; and has achieved voluntary reporting by over 670 hospitals (The Leapfrog Group 2003). Business coalitions have taken responsibility for implementing the three great leaps forward by working with their local hospitals in every site except for two. The Leapfrog Group believes that it will be business interests and not the hospital industry that will propel the industry to embrace these changes at a faster pace.

Future issues for hospital boards

Hospital board members are facing complex governance decisions in the current marketplace. Declining revenues from Medicare and Medicaid are paired with increasing numbers of uninsured. Cost increases from multiple sectors in the industry and other cost drivers have created double-digit premium increases for private payers (including hospitals in their role as employers). Payers have responded by passing increasing healthcare costs to their employees. Concurrent with declining revenues, hospital board members are now confronted with new reporting and compliance requirements by regulators, including JACHO and CMS. Attaining high-quality, affordable service is indeed a daunting task.

Hospital board members can ask some basic questions about quality of care in their institution. Examples are as follows:

- Do board members know whether their institution's morbidity, mortality, and infection rates compare favorably with their peers locally and nationally?
- Is the institution more costly because of avoidable errors? For example, are pneumonia and heart attack victims staying longer because their first doses of necessary medication occur many hours after admission instead of within the first hour?
- Does hospital leadership provide this type of information to the board or to the community?

Future directions that are likely to be embraced by coalitions and their members may include the following:

- support and encouragement of national standards and national organizations such as the National Quality Forum and the National Committee for Quality Assurance,
- development of financial and nonfinancial incentives to improve/reward high-quality healthcare,
- use of data and information to set benchmark performance requirements for hospitals and other sectors in healthcare,
- dissemination of this information to encourage wise purchasing and utilization decisions by businesses and by their employee; and
- improvement of performance and safety in the provision of healthcare services and the encouragement of continuous quality improvement.

Business coalitions are formed to lower healthcare costs to their members. In pursuit of this goal, they are dealing with local hospital leadership about both cost and quality. It is certainly the goal of both hospital boards and business coalitions to ensure the highest quality and most affordable hospital services for the benefit of all.

Notes

1. In 1987, the Joint Commission on Accreditation of Healthcare Organizations first announced the *Agenda for Change*, which outlined a series of major steps designed to modernize the accreditation process. A key component of the *Agenda for Change* was the integration of performance measurement data into the accreditation process through the implementation of the ORYX initiative. The introduction of standardized core performance measures into the ORYX initiative in 2002 will, for the first time ever, permit rigorous comparison of the actual results of care across hospitals. For more information, go to the JCAHO web site at www.jcaho.org.
2. Interested hospitals should contact IHI directly at www.IHI.org to arrange for receipt of information about their specific HSMR and strategies to "Move Your Dot."
3. Multiple web sites publish hospital-specific information. One of the more widely accessed commercial sites that provides a variety of comparative hospital information is www.healthgrades.com.

Acknowledgments

The author would like to thank the following for their contributions to this chapter: Michael Pugh, principal, Pugh Ettinger McCarthy, Pueblo, Colorado, for "What Is the Board's Role in Monitoring Quality of Healthcare?"; Cathy Barry-Ipema, chief communications officer, Joint Commission on Accreditation of Healthcare Organizations, Oakbrook Terrace, Illinois, for "What Should the Board Know About the Joint Commission on Accreditation of Healthcare Organizations?"; and Donna Marshall, executive director, Colorado Business Group on Health, Denver, for "What Should the Board Know About Business Coalitions on Health?"

References

Instititue of Medicine Committee on Quality Health Care in America. 2001. *Crossing the Quality Chasm: A New Health Care System for the 21st Century*. Washington, DC: National Academy Press.

Institute of Medicine. 2000. *To Err Is Human: Building a Safer Health System*. Washington, DC: Committee on Quality of Health Care in America, Institute of Medicine.

Joint Commission on Accreditation of Healthcare Organizations. 2003. "Facts About American Nurses Credentialing Center Magnet Recognition Program." [Online information; retrieved 6/27/03.] www.jcaho.org/news+room/press+kits/facts+about+magnet+hospitals.htm.

Kaplan, R. S., and D. P. Norton. 1996. *The Balanced Scorecard: Translating Strategy into Action*. Boston: Harvard Business School Press.

Midwest Business Group on Health. 2001. *Reducing the Costs of Poor Quality Health Care Through Responsible Purchasing Leadership*. Chicago: Midwest Business Group on Health.

National Business Coalition on Health. 2000. "NNCH Member Profile." [Online information; retrieved 6/26/03.] www.nbch.org/members.htm.

The Leapfrog Group. 2003. "About Us." [Online information; retrieved 6/26/03.] www.leapfroggroup.org/about.htm.

Suggested Resources

Agency for Healthcare Research and Quality (www.talkingquality.gov)

Centers for Medicare and Medicaid Services (www.cms.gov)

Joint Commission on Accreditation of Healthcare Organizations (www.jcaho.org)

Midwest Business Group on Health (www.mbgh.org)

National Business Coalition on Health (www.nbch.org)

National Committee for Quality Assurance (www.ncqa.org)

National Quality Forum (www.qualityforum.org)

Pacific Business Group on Health (www.healthscope.org)

CHAPTER FOUR

Fiscal Responsibility and Oversight

What Should the Board Know About Financial Oversight?

...or, Who's Minding the Checkbook?

Overall, the board has a responsibility for ensuring the organization's financial health. To do this, management and the board must work closely together in several areas. The board will approve financial objectives developed by management and the finance committee. Management needs to prepare financial statements that can be understood by all members of the board. The board has to agree on certain financial ratios that will be helpful in understanding the financial statements. The finance committee and management will look at more detailed financial ratios, but board members need to know the key parts that make up financial statements and the key financial ratios.

Use of financial statements

Financial statements issued by healthcare organizations provide useful information to internal and external decision makers. The primary financial statements—the balance sheet, the income statement, and the cash flow statement—present a summary of the results of operations and financial status for one or more time periods. The following is a more formal approach to analyzing financial statements that will provide insights into the healthcare organization's financial condition. The hospital financial statements are used to illustrate the various analytic techniques. Before delving further into specific analytic ratios, we first discuss some of the conceptual objectives of the balance sheet, income statement, and statement of cash flows.

The balance sheet. One use of the balance sheet is to provide information about the *liquidity* of the organization. The balance sheet lists the current values of cash and other cash equivalents such as certificates of deposit and marketable securities (see Figure 4.1). Comparison of resources that can be spent versus liabilities requiring future spending helps a board assess liquidity. When bills exceed what cash balances, any organization may be facing bankruptcy or other major changes. In more elegant accounting terminology, when current liabilities are greater than current assets, an organization's liquidity is severely impaired. When liquidity suffers, the risk of bankruptcy or the need for an infusion of more funds is critical.

Another use of the balance sheet is to report the net book values of fixed and other long-term assets. This portion of the balance sheet refers to the un-amortized or un-depreciated long-term assets. Since many of these values are reported at outdated or obsolete amounts, the balance sheet does not usually achieve its objective to provide useful information about the organization's long-term assets. In other words, the reader cannot determine how long the assets might continue to be used. The net book value of assets is only a proxy for the value or future benefits of such long-term assets. As long as the assets are not fully depreciated, it is assumed they will continue to provide useful, necessary, and economically efficient services. This assumption is not always justified. Since current market values are not reported on the balance sheet, the astute board member must ask questions about possible changes in market values. Users of balance sheets must know where to look for different types of information and how it can be used.

A third use of the balance sheet concerns the amounts and relative timing associated with debts and other liabilities. How much debt is due? This relates to liquidity in identifying debt payments that must be made. On an overall basis, this is called *debt management*. On the whole, most balance

Figure 4.1: Community General Hospital Balance Sheet

Year ended	12/31/03	12/31/04
Assets		
Current Assets:		
Cash	$150,000	$275,000
Marketable securities	1,039,000	1,214,000
Accounts receivable	12,072,000	4,295,000
Less allowances for doubtful accounts	(3,899,000)	(4,529,000)
Net accounts receivable	$8,173,000	$9,766,000
Supplies inventory	910,000	1,035,000
Prepaid expenses	565,000	600,000
Total current assets:	10,837,000	12,890,000
Assets limited as to use, net of amounts required to meet current obligations	0	0
Property and Equipment	57,774,950	61,013,373
Less accumulated depreciation	(25,550,621)	(30,243,852)
Net property and equipment	32,224,329	30,769,521
Other assets	20,178,412	26,864,858
Total assets:	**$63,239,741**	**$70,524,379**
Liabilities and Net Assets		
Current Liabilities:		
Accounts payable	$2,417,000	$2,275,000
Notes payable	520,000	612,000
Current portion of long-term debt	346,877	349,155
Accrued salaries	2,858,000	3,369,000
Other current liabilities	1,050,000	1,050,000
Total current liabilities:	7,191,877	7,655,155
Long-term Debt:		
Mortgage payable	4,927,037	4,580,160
Less current maturities	(346,877)	(349,155)
Net long-term debt	4,580,160	4,231,005
Equity:		
Net assets, unrestricted	51,467,704	58,638,219
Total liabilities and net assets:	**$63,239,741**	**$70,524,379**

Source: Neumann, B. 1999. *Financial Management: Concepts and Applications for Health Care Organizations*, 4th edition. Ft. Collins, CO: Kendall/Hunt Publishing Company. Adapted with permission.

sheets provide useful information about the amounts of outstanding liabilities. An assessment of relative amounts and trends in debt provides much useful information about risk and future liquidity concerns.

A final use of the balance sheet addresses how much might be left over. The *equity* section of the balance sheet includes invested capital and retained earnings, called net assets or fund balances for nonprofit organizations. This section may be viewed, in entirety, as a set of residual claims on the organization's net assets. Since this final section of the balance sheet reflects residual interests, it is used primarily to analyze the difference between assets and liabilities.

The equity section of the balance sheet does not provide any indication of market values nor does it indicate how much cash might be available if the firm's assets were sold. It only provides an indicator of relative equity interests. This is often misunderstood and may be misleading because changes in this section of the balance sheet often lag far behind the real changes that occur in real estate and other external market values.

The income statement. One of the major purposes of a for-profit organization's income statement is to provide *indicators of profitability*. Most commercial organizations exist to make money. As we have shown earlier, nonprofit organizations focus on increases or decreases in net assets. Healthcare organizations exist to improve people's wellness and cure their illness. In actual financial statements, the terms "net profit," "net income," and "increases in net assets" are slightly modified to suit each preparer's preferences. Negative income or a decrease in net assets is a loss ("red ink" in an earlier era).

The income statement is the primary source of information about profits and other changes affecting equities. In addition, income statements usually contain information about operations for one or two prior periods. Profit or net income is usually indicated under operating income on the income statement (see Figure 4.2). In fact, many readers only look at the income statement's bottom line and compare this limited view of profitability to the bottom line for other organizations. Astute board members must not take a bottom-line orientation; instead, they must look carefully at various parts of the income statement and know how profits may or may not be influenced by other indicators in the financial statements.

Figure 4.2: Community General Hospital Income Statement

Year ended	*12/31/03*	*12/31/04*
Unrestricted Revenue, Gains, and Other Support:		
Net inpatient revenue	$78,345,560	$92,573,914
Net outpatient revenue	7,843,175	9,267,576
Net patient service revenue	86,188,735	101,841,490
Other service revenues	1,609,608	1,770,569
Total revenues, gains, and other revenues:	87,798,343	103,612,059
Operating Expenses:		
Salaries	44,403,200	52,339,563
Fringe benefits	6,852,136	8,695,810
Fees	2,253,412	2,540,480
Supplies	12,024,161	13,974,551
Utilities	2,394,266	2,921,055
Provision for bad debt	7,422,553	9,161,125
Depreciation	4,029,549	4,693,531
Interest	454,003	423,721
Other expenses:	3,776,359	4,191,758
Less Total expenses:	83,609,639	98,941,544
Operating income:	4,188,704	4,670,515
Plus contributions from foundation	2,079,000	2,427,000
Increase in unrestricted net assets:	**$6,267,704**	**$7,097,515**
Per diem inpatient revenue	$905.73	$1,035.07
Per diem operating income	$48.42	$52.22
Patient days	86,500	89,437

Source: Neumann, B. 1999. *Financial Management: Concepts and Applications for Health Care Organizations,* 4th edition. Ft. Collins, CO: Kendall/Hunt Publishing Company. Adapted with permission.

To accomplish this broader purpose, consider *assessing risk* using the income statement. A clinic that has quite stable and acceptable levels of income or profit may be considered as low risk. On the other hand, a hospital with high profits one year and losses the next exhibits much higher risk. Considering the variability and volatility of information in the income statement permits the reader to better understand the level of risk, uncertainty, or unpredictability that may be encountered in the future. Any organization that exhibits high levels of fluctuations in income may experience similar levels of variations in the future.

Risk assessment goes hand-in-hand with *assessing predictability*. Reading the income statement and interpreting all of its many nuances is of little value unless some predictions about the future can be made. This may seem like fortunetelling, but it is essential to develop some future-oriented skills. By understanding prior income statements, board members should be able to predict something about what future income statements may contain. By knowing more about prior profits, members should be able to make some predictions about future profits.

Most managers and board members make these predictions on a subjective and intuitive basis. This is an art and requires much creative insight and many years of experience. For now, just remember that an income statement is of little value unless it permits some prediction of future profits. In summary, the income statement should provide information about income and changes in income.

Statement of cash flows. The cash flow statement provides similar information. For example, the cash flow statement is certainly concerned with liquidity. Have the cash flows been managed effectively and in such a way that the organization's bills are paid on a timely basis? The cash flow statement provides a vivid and easily understood indication of changes in cash balances and suggests reasons for why they have changed (see Figure 4.3).

In similar fashion, the cash flow statement addresses asset management as it summarizes the year's investing activities. Investing activities are usually intended to maintain or achieve shifts in the organization's operating capabilities. As a separate section of the cash flow statement, all of the year's investing activities are clearly disclosed. Therefore, the cash flow statement is one of the best ways to assess how assets are being used or replaced.

Likewise, the cash flow statement has a separate section on financing activities, which relates to the debt management. Since the cash flow statement summarizes all changes in long-term debt, it is an excellent source for examining how managers might be changing their debt management strategies by obtaining more debt or reducing debt. While managers might not explicitly disclose such strategies, they often become apparent when cash flow statements for several periods are compared and analyzed.

Figure 4.3: Community General Hospital Cash Flow Statement (abbreviated direct method)

Year ended	12/31/03	12/31/04
Operating Activities:		
Collection from patients	$85,096,753	$102,019,057
Payments to employees	(43,982,200)	(51,828,563)
Other operating activities	(36,416,021)	(44,813,701)
Cash Provided by Operating Activities:	4,698,514	5,376,793
Financing Activities:		
Contributions	2,079,000	2,427,000
Incur (redeem long-term debt)	(346,887)	(349,155)
Cash provided by financing activities	1,732,113	2,077,845
Investing Activities:		
Purchase "other assets"	(2,906,038)	(6,686,446)
Purchase land, buildings, and equipment	(1,981,589)	1,454,808
Cash Used in Investing Activities:	(4,887,627)	(5,231,638)
Annual Increase in Cash:	**$1,543,000**	**$2,223,000**
Example:		
Cash provided by operating activities	$4,698,514	$5,376,793
+ Cash provided by financing activities	$1,732,113	$2,077,845
- Cash used in investing activities	($4,887,627)	(5,231,638)
= Annual increase in cash	$1,543,000	$2,223,000

Source: Neumann, B. 1999. *Financial Management: Concepts and Applications for Health Care Organizations*, 4th edition. Ft. Collins, CO: Kendall/Hunt Publishing Company. Adapted with permission.

Use of financial ratios

The magnitude of data presented in typical financial statements makes it difficult to formulate judgments about the financial condition of an organization without further analysis. For example, Figures 4.1 through 4.3 present two years of financial statements for a nonprofit hospital, Community General Hospital. These statements illustrate the typical financial analysis techniques that can be applied to either for-profit or nonprofit organizations. Effective analysis of these statements requires systematic ratio analysis.

A ratio expresses the relationship between two numbers, such as current assets and current liabilities. Unfortunately, by itself, a single ratio calculation is difficult to evaluate, unless some standards or normative values are available for comparative purposes. Comparisons with industry norms and comparisons with prior ratio values in the same organization can provide useful insight. We will concentrate on historical comparisons.

For example, the current ratio is commonly computed as the relationship between current assets and current liabilities (current ratio = current assets/ current liabilities). This ratio is then used to make judgments about the ability of an organization to meet its short-term obligations. From the 2004 data for Community General Hospital in Figure 4.1, a current ratio of 1.68 can be computed (12,890,000 / 7,655,155 = 1.68). Using a single data point for 2004 is somewhat problematic. However, when the ratio for the previous year is computed, a different evaluation might be made. The current ratio for 2003 is 1.51. This represents a positive trend, and it appears that the management of Community General is improving its liquidity.

The use of ratio analysis as a management tool requires some caution for several reasons. First, definitions for the same ratio may vary. Thus, the analyst must document which definition is used and must interpret the results accordingly. In this section, we use common definitions, but alternatives are available. Second, finding a comparison group that matches a provider in all aspects is difficult. Third, since some leeway is allowed in preparing financial statements in accordance with generally accepted accounting principles, different balance sheet valuations can influence the ratio results. Finally, interpretation of the ratios often involves judgment. Different board members may interpret the same results somewhat differently.

Ratio categories. Ratios are used to facilitate evaluation of the financial condition of an organization. This evaluation is most effective when similar ratios are used to reflect management decisions or strategies.

- *Liquidity ratios* focus primarily on the balance sheet and help assess how the organization manages its short-term liquidity and its working capital.
- *Turnover ratios* use data from both the balance sheet and the income statement. They facilitate the analysis of efficiency ratios, using the

income statement as a measure of outputs and the balance sheet as a measure of inputs. Collectively, liquidity ratios, capitalization ratios, and turnover ratios help a board member make informed judgments about the healthcare organization's financial condition and performance.

- *Profitability ratios* generally use data from the income statement and are sometimes called performance ratios because they summarize the primary dimensions of an organization's fiscal and financial performance, generally linking the income statement and the balance sheet.

- *Capitalization ratios* also focus primarily on the balance sheet and permit an examination of long-term financing strategies, including the amount of long-term debt financing, changes in capital structure, and the ability to repay existing long-term debt.

Each of these four commonly used ratio categories is presented more specifically below. One technical caveat must be noted: wherever the term "cash" is indicated, all forms of cash and cash equivalents are intended.

1. Liquidity

$$\text{Current Ratio} = \frac{\text{Current assets}}{\text{Current liabilities}}$$

(Measures extent to which current obligations can be covered by current assets)

$$\text{Quick Ratio} = \frac{\text{Cash + Net accounts receivable + Marketable securities}}{\text{Current liabilities}}$$

(Represents a more stringent definition of current assets)

$$\text{Acid Test Ratio} = \frac{\text{Cash + Marketable securities}}{\text{Current liabilities}}$$

(Reflects the composition of current assets, recognizing that accounts receivable and inventories, although current assets, cannot be expended to cover current liabilities)

$$\text{Cushion Ratio} = \frac{\text{Cash + Marketable Securities + Board-designated restricted cash}}{\text{Annual Debt Service}}$$

(Includes cash, other short-term investments, and cash in board-designated accounts and ties the balance sheet and income statement together)

$$\text{Daily Cash Flow} = \frac{\text{Operating expenses - (depreciation + other noncash charges)}}{\text{Days in period}}$$

(Shows how much cash is needed to sustain operations on a daily basis)

$$\text{Days of Cash Available} = \frac{\text{Cash}}{\text{Daily cash flow}}$$

(Indicates the real margin of safety for the hospital. The hospital should have one pay-roll period of days cash flow available)

2. Turnover Ratios

$$\text{Total Asset Turnover} = \frac{\text{Total Revenues}}{\text{Total Assets}}$$

(Measures the amount of revenue generated by each dollar of capital investment)

$$\text{Accounts Receivable Turnover} = \frac{\text{Net patient service revenue}}{\text{Net accounts receivable}}$$

(Indicates how often each year accounts receivable are recycled into patient revenue)

Average Collection Period = 365 days/accounts receivable turnover

(Measures number of days in average collection period. This and above ratio are related)

$$\text{Average Accounts Payable Turnover} = \frac{\text{Cost of supplies}}{\text{Accounts payable}}$$

(This ratio and the next one measure number of days usage and length of the payment period. These ratios are measures of solvency that uses adjusted current liabilities in the computations)

$$\text{Accounts Payable Period} = \frac{365}{\text{accounts payable turnover}}$$

$$\text{Inventory Turnover} = \frac{\text{Cost of supplies}}{\text{Supplies inventory}}$$

(Measures efficiency of hospital's inventory—that is the amount of revenue generated by each dollar invested in inventory)

3. Profitability Ratios

$$\text{Operating Margin} = \frac{\text{Operating income}}{\text{Total revenues}}$$

(Measures profitability [e.g., reflects the proportion of operating revenue retained as income])

$$\text{Return on Assets} = \frac{\text{Increase in unrestricted net assets (or net income)}}{\text{Total assets}}$$

(Measures the dollars of income generated for every dollar invested in assets)

$$\text{Return on Equity} = \frac{\text{Increase in unrestricted net assets (or net income)}}{\text{Net assets}}$$

(Measures the amount of patient service revenues that are lost to uncollected accounts receivable)

$$\text{Bad Debt Ratio} = \frac{\text{Provision for bad debt}}{\text{Net patient service revenue}}$$

(Measures the amount of patient service revenues that are lost to uncollected accounts receivable)

4. Capitalization Ratios

$$\text{Long-term Debt to Total Assets Ratio} = \frac{\text{Long-term debt}}{\text{Total assets}}$$

(Looks at long-term debt in the hospital capital structure. High values increases the difficulty and expense associated with securing long-term in the future)

$$\text{Days of Cash Available} = \frac{\text{Cash}}{\text{Daily cash flow}}$$

(Indicates the real margin of safety for the hospital. The hospital should have one payroll period of days cash flow available)

$$\text{Times Interest Earned} = \frac{\text{Operating Income + Interest expense}}{\text{Interest expense}}$$

(Evaluates the ability to pay existing debt payments)

Debt Service Coverage =

$$\frac{\text{Operating income} + \text{Depreciation expense} + \text{Annual debt service requirements}}{\text{Annual debt service requirements}}$$

(Measure of the organization's ability to pay its long-term debt)

Average Age of Plant = $\dfrac{\text{Accumulated depreciation}}{\text{Depreciation expense}}$

(A measure of the number of years of depreciation that have been expensed and is an indicator of the need to replace and/or renovate the physical plant)

Illustration: Community General Hospital

The financial statements of Community General Hospital, presented in Figures 4.1 through 4.3, are similar to the financial statements issued by many nonprofit hospitals. To illustrate the basic elements of financial analysis, ratios are computed for Community General using those financial statements. Although a hospital is used in the sample illustrations, the same methods could be used in analyzing the financial statements of any healthcare organization. The importance of different ratios will vary for different types of organizations.

Liquidity ratios. Perhaps the ratio most frequently used to reflect short-term liquidity is the *current ratio*. It relates current assets to current liabilities and is useful in identifying possible short-run financial problems.

The term *current assets* is usually interpreted to mean those assets that will be converted to cash in less than one year. Similarly, *current liabilities* are those liabilities that are to be paid within one year. A current ratio greater than one (1.0) is considered a sign of prudent fiscal management, for this allows a margin of safety in the ability to meet current obligations. Based on the 2003–2004 trends in its current ratios, it appears that Community General has been slowly improving its management of current assets and current liabilities. Many firms operate successfully with current ratios that are close to 1.0. Therefore, Community General's current ratio may reflect prudent management of current assets and could minimize the cost of holding them. However, it may also reflect a narrow margin of safety to meet current liabilities. Should cash flow be reduced for any reason, alternative sources of funds such as short-term financing may be needed on short notice to meet current obligations.

$$\text{Current Ratio} = \frac{\text{Current assets}}{\text{Current liabilities}}$$

2003: $\dfrac{10{,}837{,}000}{7{,}191{,}877} = 1.51$ **2004:** $\dfrac{12{,}890{,}000}{7{,}755{,}155} = 1.68$

To further assess liquidity, many analysts also compute a *quick ratio*. The quick ratio represents a more stringent definition of current assets, as only cash, net patient accounts receivable, and marketable securities are considered available to meet current liabilities.

$$\text{Quick Ratio} = \frac{\text{Cash + Net patient accounts receivable + Marketable securities}}{\text{Current liabilities}}$$

2003: $\dfrac{150{,}000 + 8{,}173{,}000 + 1{,}039{,}000}{7{,}191{,}877} = 1.30$

2004: $\dfrac{275{,}000 + 9{,}766{,}000 + 1{,}214{,}000}{7{,}655{,}155} = 1.47$

The quick ratios for Community General also indicate an improvement in the liquidity position over the two years as noted.

A more focused liquidity ratio is called the *acid test ratio*. The acid test ratio includes only "spendable" resources because marketable securities can be turned into cash very quickly.

$$\text{Acid Test Ratio} = \frac{\text{Cash + Marketable securities}}{\text{Current liabilities}}$$

2003: $\dfrac{150.000 + 1{,}039{,}000}{7{,}191{,}877} = 1.17$ **2004:** $\dfrac{275{,}000 + 1{,}214{,}000}{7{,}655{,}155} = 0.19$

Community General's acid test ratios are quite stable. One might expect more volatility in this ratio unless cash balances are managed at year end to achieve certain targets. For example, an organization may try to show high cash balances at the end of the year as a safety measure or to instill confidence in potential investors.

To summarize, all three liquidity ratios (current, quick, and acid test) indicate that Community General is increasing current assets in relation to its current liabilities. If a firm has easy access to short-term debt or other sources of short-term funds, then a relatively low liquidity position will tend to minimize the costs associated with managing current assets. In other words, the funds that would have been used to provide liquidity can be used to provide other, perhaps more essential, patient services. If alternative short-term sources of funding are not available, and some major payers delay payment for any reason, Community General could find itself in a cash bind. The increasing trend in these ratios may indicate that management has been making a concerted effort to improve its liquidity position.

A variety of cash-based ratios might also be calculated to further assess the hospital's liquidity. Many cash ratios rely on data from the statement of cash flows (Figure 4.3). One of the more interesting cash ratios is the *cushion ratio* used by Standard & Poor (S & P) in determining its credit ratings. S&P generally expects the cushion ratio to exceed 6.0.

The cushion ratio is interesting on several counts because it includes cash and other short-term investments (marketable securities and other cash equivalents) and cash in board-designated accounts (which may have otherwise been ignored in a liquidity analysis), and it ties the balance sheet and income statement together. The numerator emphasizes substance over form and should include all forms of liquid, spendable cash, or cash equivalents.

In general, cushion ratios should emphasize and include terms that are defined on a substance-over-form basis (i.e., include all similar items that properly reflect liquidity or profitability that are a focus of that ratio). In many cases, it is instructive to compute the ratio first using a narrow definition of the terms, and, second, to compute the same ratio using much broader and more inclusive definitions.

To get a complete understanding of an organization's cushion ratio, one might calculate it first as indicated above, using only internally restricted liquid assets, and then include all liquid assets, some of which might be restricted by donors. This second calculation might also extend the entity definition to include related foundations or other closely controlled affiliates. In other words, the substance-over-form question requires the analyst to look for other sources of liquidity that may be controlled by the healthcare organization.

In the denominator of the cushion ratio, two financial statements are tied together where the annual interest expense is added to the annual principal repayments on long-term debt. Sometimes, the annual debt service is shown in the notes to the financial statements. In other cases, the annual

principal payments must be estimated. Principal payments can also sometimes be found on the cash flow statement. What is most interesting about
the denominator is that there is no single source where annual debt service
can always be found. The astute analyst must often piece together the various elements or estimate them.

To calculate annual debt service, find the interest expense on the income
statement and the payments on long-term debt or the current maturities of
long-term debt on the balance sheet. In our example, we use the current portion of long-term debt from the balance sheet. We use the interest expense
from the current income statement; however, more correctly, we should use
the actual interest paid if that figure is available.

Annual Debt Service = Interest expense + Annual principal payments

$$\text{Cushion Ratio} = \frac{\text{Cash + Marketable securities + Board-designated restricted cash}}{\text{Annual debt service}}$$

2003: $\dfrac{150.000 + 1,039,000 + 0}{454,003 + 346,877} = \dfrac{1,189,000}{800,880} = 1.48$

2004: $\dfrac{275,000 + 1,214,000 + 0}{423,721 + 349,155} = \dfrac{1,489,000}{772,876} = 1.93$

Turnover ratios. One of management's primary responsibilities is the efficient use of assets. Turnover or activity ratios can provide useful information in this area. Data from both the balance sheet and the income statement are needed to compute turnover ratios.

The *total asset turnover ratio* is a key indicator of how efficiently assets are
being used to generate revenues. This ratio shows the amount of revenue obtained from each dollar of assets.

$$\text{Total asset turnover ratio} = \frac{\text{Total revenues, gains, and other support}}{\text{Total assets}}$$

2003: $\dfrac{87,798,343}{63,329,741} = 1.39$ **2004:** $\dfrac{103,612,069}{70,524,379} = 1.47$

Community General appears to be making excellent use of its assets to
create revenue. Any result greater than 1.0 for this ratio implies that management is monitoring investments in assets relatively closely and maxi-
mizing the assets' ability to generate revenues.

Another highly informative turnover ratio is the *accounts receivable turnover ratio* and its related statistic, the *average collection period*. These are the primary ratios tracked by experienced healthcare managers in provider firms, mainly because of the size of the investment in receivables at most hospitals and the often lengthy collection periods from third-party payers. Managed care organizations and other payers would not be as concerned about accounts receivable because they receive their funds regularly each month in the form of premiums or other contractual payments.

$$\frac{\text{Accounts Receivable Turnover}}{\text{(A/R Turnover)}} = \frac{\text{Net patient services revenue}}{\text{Net accounts receivable}}$$

2003: $\dfrac{86,188,735}{8,173,000} = 10.55$ **2004:** $\dfrac{101,841,490}{9,766,000} = 10.43$

$$\frac{\text{Average Collection Period}}{\text{(in days)}} = \frac{365 \text{ days}}{\text{Accounts receivable turnover}}$$

2003: $\dfrac{365 \text{ days}}{10.55} = 34.60 \text{ days}$ **2004:** $\dfrac{365 \text{ days}}{10.43} = 35.00 \text{ days}$

Overall, Community General's average collection period is excellent; however, the decreasing trend in accounts receivable turnover, which results in a slight increasing trend in the average collection period, might be of some concern to management. It may mean that collection procedures are becoming lax, a different type of patient is being served, or the major third-party purchasers (payers) are changing their payment policies.

A similar approach to the accounts receivable computations can be used for accounts payable, inventory, and current assets. The number of days' usage in each category and the length of the payment period can identify potential problems before they become serious and result in poor vendor relationships. For example, with respect to accounts payable, the *accounts payable turnover* and *accounts payable payment period* are:

$$\frac{\text{Accounts Payable Turnover}}{\text{(A/P Turnover)}} = \frac{\text{Cost of supplies}}{\text{Accounts payable}}$$

2003: $\dfrac{12,204,161}{2,417,000} = 4.97$ **2004:** $\dfrac{13,974,551}{2,275,000} = 6.14$

$$\frac{\text{Accounts Payable Payment Period}}{\text{(in days)}} = \frac{365 \text{ days}}{\text{Accounts receivable turnover}}$$

2003: $\dfrac{365 \text{ days}}{4.97} = 73.44 \text{ days}$ **2004:** $\dfrac{365 \text{ days}}{6.14} = 59.45 \text{ days}$

Community General seems to be doing an excellent job of utilizing its assets. Its total asset turnover ratio is high and its average collection period for accounts receivable is very good. However, two possible areas of concern include the slight change in the average collection period and the slow payment to vendors for supplies. The long accounts payable cycle is in keeping with Community General's low current ratio and helps the cash flow by delaying payment as much as possible. However, the slow payment for supplies could strain vendor relationships since most vendors allow only 30 days before payment is due. If Community General were to run into liquidity problems in the future and need additional time to make payments, its creditors may not be very receptive.

The *inventory turnover ratio* is analogous to both accounts receivable and accounts payable turnover ratios. It measures the efficiency of the hospital's inventory management practices.

Profitability ratios. Profitability ratios provide a more global perspective to performance evaluation of healthcare organizations. They indicate how much better off the organization is as a result of profits or changes in net assets. Two closely related ratios are the operating margin and the return on assets.

The *operating margin ratio* expresses the difference between the revenues received from providing services and the expenses required to support these revenues as a percentage of total revenues. We use operating income, or excess of revenues over expenses, in the numerator of this ratio because it most clearly expresses the financial impact of "core business" operations, as compared to other sources of funds that may be shown elsewhere on the income statement. However, some analysts may prefer to use net income (or change in net assets) as the numerator in this ratio. When net income is used, the ratio is called the net income ratio.

Operating Margin = $\dfrac{\text{Operating income}}{\text{Total revenues}}$

2003: $\dfrac{4,188,704}{87,798,343} = 0.048$ 　　　　　　　　**2004:** $\dfrac{4,670,515}{103,612,059} = 0.045$

$\dfrac{\text{Return on Assets}}{\text{(ROA)}} = \dfrac{\text{Increase in unrestricted net assets (or net income)}}{\text{Total assets}}$

2003: $\dfrac{6,267,704}{63,239,741} = 0.099$ 　　　　　　　　**2004:** $\dfrac{7,097,515}{70,524,379} = 0.101$

The *return on assets ratio* expresses the net income (increase in unrestricted net assets) as a percentage of the assets employed to provide services or products. This is an overall profitability ratio because it uses the bottom line on the income statement. Both operating margin and return on assets ratios provide managers with a perspective on how revenues, expenses, and assets were used to provide healthcare services or products. If the operating margin is too low, management has the option of raising prices or reducing expenses. Either alternative would result in an increase in the operating margin. If the return on assets is low, management can either increase the operating margin as indicated above or reduce the amount of assets utilized.

The return on assets for Community General is very good, but the declining trends may indicate a potential problem. The declining operating margin may be due to a number of factors, including an increase in government sponsored or managed care patients where the hospital is paid at discounted rates. However, the declining operating margin may indicate that management is not raising rates fast enough. Another possible explanation might include inefficient or costly operations. Many factors contribute to positive and negative operating margins, and these profitability ratios are summary measures of many interrelated factors.

Another ratio commonly used to diagnose profitability is the *bad debt ratio*. This ratio measures the amount of patient service revenues lost to uncollected accounts receivable. In our example, we compare bad debt expenses to net patient service revenue (an alternative is to calculate separate bad debt ratios for inpatient or outpatient revenue).

$$\text{Bad debt ratio} = \frac{\text{Provision for bad debts}}{\text{Net patient service revenue}}$$

2003: $\dfrac{7,422,553}{86,188,735} = 0.086$ **2004:** $\dfrac{9,161,125}{101,841,490} = 0.090$

Bad debts are fairly stable ratio, indicating that the collection procedures used to manage bad debts have been effective. One final profitability ratio is the *return on equity ratio*, which shows the returns on investment (ROI).

Capitalization ratios. The final group of ratios concentrates on capital structure and ability to pay long-term debt. These ratios help evaluate the organization's financial flexibility and the amount of risk associated with debt financing. Another commonly used term for this group of ratios is *leverage ratios*. Basically, *financial leverage* refers to why hospitals might incur more debt as compared to other sources of financing. Leverage analysis usually assumes that debt is less costly, such that having more debt will reduce the organization's financing costs. Increasing proportions of debt usually means reduced flexibility in obtaining future financing (further lending may not be available) and increased risks (due to increased variability in net income). When the proportion of debt in the organization's capital structure becomes too high, lenders may also increase the cost of debt (interest expense).

The *long-term debt to total assets ratio* is one way of evaluating debt management policies. The long-term debt to total assets ratio shows trends in how debt has been used. The second major indicator of financial risk associated with capitalization is the *times-interest-earned ratio*, which evaluates the ability to pay existing debt payments. We use operating income, or excess of revenues over expenses, in the numerator of this ratio because it most closely approximates the sustainable, or long-term, income flows that can be expected in the future. Since the times-interest-earned ratio is a proxy for risk, we are most interested in how this ratio is likely to evolve in the future. The major capitalization ratios for Community General are as follows:

$$\text{Long-term Debt to Total Assets (LTD)} = \frac{\text{Long-term debts}}{\text{Total assets}}$$

2003: $\dfrac{4{,}580{,}160}{63{,}239{,}741} = 0.07$ **2004:** $\dfrac{4{,}231{,}005}{70{,}524{,}379} = 0.06$

Times-Interest-Earned (TIE) ratio $= \dfrac{\text{Operating income} + \text{Interest expense}}{\text{Interest expense}}$

2003: $\dfrac{4{,}188{,}704 + 454{,}003}{454{,}003} = 10.23$ **2004:** $\dfrac{4670{,}515 + 423{,}721}{423{,}721} = 12.02$

The long-term financial structure of Community General indicates that considerable *debt capacity* exists. If Community General sets a maximum debt capacity of 50 percent of total assets, then its long-term debt capacity in 2003 is $31,619,857 [=.5(63,239,714)]. With only $4,580,160 in long-term debt currently outstanding, Community General has $27,039,697 in additional debt capacity. This estimate of additional long-term debt capacity is reinforced by the times-interest-earned ratio of 9–23, which is quite high. It appears that Community General has considerable flexibility in its financial structure to meet future requirements and can borrow as needed on a long-term or a short-term basis.

One other capitalization ratio is the *debt service coverage ratio*. It would be calculated only in the event that other capitalization ratios indicated potential financing problems. A final ratio is the *average age of plant*, which could be an indicator of the need to replace or renovate the physical plant.

Overall assessment. The financial ratios computed for Community General indicate a healthy overall financial condition with flexibility in financing for the future. The low level of long-term debt provides the borrowing capacity that will permit Community General to take advantage of opportunities such as joint ventures, mergers, and the like. More information on the $41.5 million held in other investments would be helpful in assessing the hospital's overall financial condition. The hospital also has used its assets well to generate revenues and profits. Although its short-term liquidity has been improving, Community General's management should evaluate why it remains low. It should pay special attention to the slow payment of accounts payable.

This analysis of Community General Hospital has used only the more commonly recognized relationships. The number of ratios that can actually be computed is constrained only by the analyst's imagination. The ratios that we have illustrated are usually computed first; if questions arise, then additional ratios may be necessary. We have barely scratched the surface in terms of illustrating how financial analysis can be conducted. These techniques allow the analyst to gain better understanding and more insight into the financial performance of a healthcare organization. By calculating a few ratios, the analyst may just uncover more questions requiring additional ratio calculations tailored to the specific issue.

In summary, ratio analysis is an effective tool used by boards to pinpoint possible problem areas before they can become serious. It allows board members to concentrate their efforts on the most critical issues and helps identify areas for further attention. The availability of comparative data from national services will also make ratio analysis techniques accessible to board members in any healthcare organization.

While we have illustrated ratio techniques in the context of a nonprofit hospital, similar analyses can be applied to other healthcare providers as well as to payer organizations such as insurance companies or managed care organizations. In all cases, the reader of financial statements must be careful to understand the organization's underlying motivations and incentives. Do not be confused by a mechanical application of these techniques; instead, use them to understand the meaning and implications of the decisions underlying the financial statements.

Acknowledgment

The author would like to thank Bruce R. Neumann, PH.D., professor of accounting and health management, University of Colorado–Denver, for his contributions to this chapter.

Reference

Neumann, B. 1999. *Financial Management: Concepts and Applications for Health Care Organizations*, 4th edition. Ft. Collins, CO: Kendall/Hunt Publishing Company.

CHAPTER FIVE

Responsibility for Community Relations

What Should the Board Know About Stakeholders?

...or, Who Cares?

A hospital has various individuals and other organizations—stakeholders—interested and involved in the services it provides and how it functions. The hospital must identify and interact well with its stakeholders, or it can run the risk of failing to achieve its mission and goals.

What is stakeholder analysis, and why do it?

Effective management of today's healthcare organizations requires both a new concept of the organization (i.e., a network rather than a hierarchy) and new approaches to the practical issues and problems of the complex care environment. In the emerging network, healthcare organizations are increasingly more dependent on stakeholder relationships. Consequently, efforts must be increasingly focused on the development, maintenance, and integration of favorable working relationships with stakeholders.

Healthcare leaders must build relationships with resource-based stakeholders to maintain and enhance their ability to obtain both the intellectual/human capital and the structural capital they need to create, sustain, and enhance their organization's value-creating capacity. Examples of human/intellectual capital include physicians, nurses, and other health-related professionals. Structural capital is the knowledge that is embedded in clinical and business decision support systems, such as diagnostic algorithms, disease management guidelines, protocols, clinical pathways, actuarial formulas, and databases and information systems that codify and store the organization's knowledge. The same applies to customers (third-party payers and patients) as well as to a broad array of financial capital and physical asset and material-supplier stakeholders.

Likewise, within its industry, a healthcare organization's leadership is challenged to establish and maintain relationships that enable the organization to enhance its position in the marketplace while conforming to relevant regulatory guidelines and industry standards. Finally, in the social-political arena, a healthcare organization's leadership is challenged to identify social/political stakeholders and issues, anticipate new social/political developments, and mobilize stakeholders to respond, ensuring long-term benefits (or at least no harm) to the extended organization and its critical stakeholders.

In today's world, boards must recognize that the linkages between their extended organization and its multiple stakeholders are increasingly critical to the organization's ability to sustain and enhance its value and wealth-creating capacity. With the organization's long-term survival and success growing more dependent on stakeholder relationships, knowledge about stakeholders is a critical source of competitive advantage. It is vital for an organization's board to understand who the organization's stakeholders are, including employees, medical staffs, investors, customers (third-party payers and patients), and their various communities and other constituencies. In addition to knowing who these groups are, it is necessary to know what the values and concerns of the respective stakeholders are and, in the development and implementation of organizational policies and practices, how to take into account the goals and concerns of all relevant stakeholders. Thus, stakeholder analysis—the knowledge and understanding of an organization's stakeholders—is critical to stakeholder management.

Who might be a hospital's stakeholders?

As described above, a stakeholder is any party who either affects or is affected by the organization and its goals and objectives. An organization's stakeholders are all the individuals and constituencies, both inside and outside of the organization, who contribute either voluntarily or involuntarily to its value-creating capacity and activities and who are therefore its potential beneficiaries and/or risk bearers (Post, Preston, and Sachs 2002). Stakeholders are also those individuals and organizations who are in a position to affect the organization's adoption of strategies and/or the implementation of decisions or actions.

An organization's stakeholders can be categorized into three groups—internal, interface, and external stakeholders.

1. Internal stakeholders are those groupings of people who operate entirely within the boundaries of the organization. Examples of internal stakeholders would include the organization's management team and employees.

2. Interface stakeholders are those who function both internally and externally in relation to the organization. Examples of interface stakeholders include the medical staff and others such as joint venture partners.

3. External stakeholders fall into three categories in their relationship to the organization. Some provide inputs to the organization, some compete with it, and others have a special interest in how the organization functions.

   - Those providing inputs include members or patients, third-party payers, and equipment and material vendors.

   - Those who compete with the organization for members, patients, and resources.

   - Special interest groups are concerned with the impact of the organization's operations relative to their specific interests. Examples of interest groups include formal and informal interest groups, economic-development organizations, and governmental regulatory bodies.

Stakeholder importance, concerns, and exchange of value with the organization

Integrating a stakeholder perspective into organizational management, including board leadership decisions and activities, means the board and top management must become alert and responsive to their stakeholders' concerns and priorities. Also, their tasks in managing the organization's network of stakeholders includes identifying the respective stakeholders effect on the success or failure of the organizations; specifying the goals to be achieved in stakeholder relationships, the factors contributing to goal achievement, and the risks involved; identifying opportunities for mutual benefits; and monitoring inter-stakeholder relationships and identifying interventions to harmonize or balance them as much as possible.

The stakeholder analysis worksheet in Figure 5.1 is a tool that an organization's board leadership might use to assess the relative importance of its respective stakeholders, the stakeholders' concerns, and the mutual expectations and benefits of the respective relationships.

Organizations interested in a more in-depth assessment of the worth of a potential or existing stakeholder relationship can use the following additional questions to assess that value:

1. What resources of the organization and each of its stakeholders are of value to the other?
2. What specific benefits will accrue to each stakeholder from its relationship with the organization?
3. Do benefits outweigh the costs and risks of the relationship between the organization and the respective stakeholders?
4. What social value can be generated through the organization's relationship with the respective stakeholders?
5. What new resources, capabilities, and benefits can be created through the relationship with the respective stakeholders?
6. Are the benefits equitably balanced between the organization and its respective stakeholders?
7. Has the organization's value exchange and creation with the respective stakeholders depreciated? If so, to what extent?
8. Can the organization value construct with its respective stakeholders be renewed and enhanced?

Figure 5.1: Stakeholder Analysis Worksheet

Stakeholder: _____

1. Importance of stakeholder group
    How large is the membership of this stakeholder group? _____
    How important is this stakeholder group to the organization?
    _____ Very important
    _____ Fairly important
    _____ Neutral
    _____ Not so important
    _____ Not at all important

2. Concerns of the stakeholder group
    What social, political, economic, health, or technical issues(s) is/are the pri-
    mary concerns of the stakeholder?

    Exchange of "value" between stakeholder group and the organization
    a) Stakeholder expectations/perceptions of the organization?
        •   What does this group expect to get from the organization?
        •   How satisfied is this group with what it is getting from the
            organization?
    b) Organization's expectations/dependency on stakeholder group?
        •   What input does the organization receive from this group?
        •   To what extent is the organization dependent on this group?
        •   What does the organization expect from this group?
        •   How does this stakeholder group affect the organization's
            success or failure?

Summary

A stakeholder view and approach to management is an ongoing search for value that can be created jointly with stakeholder partners but not by the organization alone. The highest value is realized when the core capabilities and resources of both the organization and its respective stakeholders are deployed to produce benefits that cannot be obtained from any other alliance. In addition to specifying the expected benefits derived from each stakeholder relationship, the organization should also indicate the incremental social value that the relationship is expected to create. For an organization and its respective stakeholders to retain their vitality and mutual engagement, benefit flows must be two way and relatively balanced. Unlike commercial partnerships' benefits, which are often reduced to monetary terms, stakeholder relationships deal in multiple currencies, some of which are difficult to quantify. A sense of equitable reciprocity between an organization and its stakeholders is essential to ensure mutual interest in investing in the relationship.

Finally, it is important to recognize that stakeholder relationships are depreciable assets and that the value of a relationship can decline over time. Renewing value is thus an ever-present challenge in maintaining stakeholder relationships. Constant attention to the value-generation process and to identifying ways to produce mutual benefits and higher levels of social good are essential to value renewal.

What Should a Board Know About the Health Status of Its Community?

...or, Is Anybody Sick Around Here?

Boards of hospitals and other healthcare organizations should be actively monitoring the health status of their communities. They should be aware of baseline information that allows them to see if improvements are being made in the community's health status or if new problems are developing. Several hospitals have even tied the CEO's and senior management's compensation packages to measurable improvements in the health status of the community. That certainly sends a clear message to management and others that the board considers the health status of the community a major concern.

An initial community health needs assessment survey should be completed by management or a consulting firm to show the board the present health status of its community. On a hospital board, the quality and community health committee is usually responsible to the board for reviewing the community's health status and making recommendations.

A discussion of the basic components of a complete community health needs assessment survey follows.

Consumer perception, awareness, and satisfaction survey

It is important that healthcare providers obtain accurate and reliable feedback from the customer groups that are key to its quality management and service satisfaction efforts. Understanding how the community perceives the organization and/or specific services or departments is important to the organization's strategic planning and positioning efforts. Respondents should be asked a series of questions about their satisfaction with past care and services provided by the organization and any area competitors. Compilation of quality and service satisfaction data helps providers assess how they are perceived by their constituents and by the community in general.

Many organizations are also interested in determining whether respondents would be interested in new services or products. Respondents are asked to indicate how likely it would be that they or their family members would utilize a specific service or program if it became available. This type of research can reduce costs and save staff time and energy spent on new product development. During this portion of the study, respondents are also often asked if they are aware that the organization offers certain programs and services. Low awareness may indicate that the organization should increase its marketing efforts to improve or increase utilization of certain programs and services.

General health indicators study/health profile

A comprehensive assessment of the community's morbidity and mortality data should be conducted. Epidemiological data are analyzed and evaluated to determine major causes of death and illness in the community. Morbidity, mortality, and demographic data are compared to state and national data, and similarities and variances are identified and analyzed. Some communities have much lower or higher incidence of mortality and morbidity from certain diseases. Knowing what illnesses are affecting the health and longevity of the organization's community is critical to service planning and development. The types of data collected from secondary sources include demographic data, health status indicators, perinatal indicators, mortality data, morbidity data, and sociodemographic indicators.

Population-wide patterns of health services use and health needs assessment

Information about population-wide patterns of use and care needs is collected, usually through telephone surveys of randomly selected members in the target area. These surveys are designed to identify issues associated with access, affordability, and availability of healthcare services and to obtain information about the healthcare needs of the population and patterns of healthcare service use, participation in risky lifestyles, and knowledge of managed care programs and insurance. The healthcare organization can then use this information to develop preventative health services and programs with the objectives of improving the overall health and well-being of the community. This type of research methodology also involves reviewing health provider assessments, diagnosed and self-reported disease, lifestyle risk factors, and demographic identifiers.

Community health needs assessment

Upon completion of the consumer perceptions and awareness survey, the general health indicators study/health profile, and the population-wide health services use and health needs assessment, a comprehensive report should be submitted to management (if management did not conduct them) and to the quality and community health committee of the board. The report should provide an analysis of all studies and synthesize results into a series of conclusions and recommendations. Based on the findings, management and/or the quality and community health committee will make recommendations to the board regarding new service or program development, community perceptions and attitudes about care, and community health needs activities and address key strategic planning issues. The board's job is to review highlights and key indicators of improvement in the community's health status, as surveyed by management and the quality and community health committee, and to act on the recommendations.

Acknowledgment

The author would like to thank Kenneth Bopp, PH.D., clinical professor, director, Health Management and Informatics Group, University of Missouri, Columbia, for his contribution of the "What Should the Board Know About Stakeholders?" section of this chapter.

Reference

Post, J. E., L. E. Preston, and S. Sachs. 2002. "Managing the Extended Enterprise: The New Stakeholder View." *California Management Review* 45 (1): 6–28.

CHAPTER SIX

Formation and Structure of a Board

What Is the Optimum Size for a Board?

...or, The Goldilocks Question: Are We Too Big or Too Small?

Does the size of your board help or hinder getting the proper things done? This is a question facing many boards in this age of increased stress in healthcare. The expectations to a board addressing its size involve county, district, and city hospitals, which have essentially no say in their size, as that has been determined by their creating authorities.

Most nonprofit boards tend to be larger than they should be, having grown too quickly in their early formative years. Historically, hospitals wanted to retain support from as many stakeholder groups as possible; a seat on the board provided concrete evidence of the esteem the hospital had for the stakeholder group. Likewise, many hospitals wanted to have as many potential donors as possible; representation from major community corporations brought those corporations into the hospital's family. Some hospitals also wanted geographic representation, particularly if they provided care in a large service area in a county or several counties.

However, in today's world, the board must look critically at membership in terms of what is needed for the good of the organization, not as a reward or incentive to contribute.

Although each board will need to determine its own magic number, as a general starting point, boards of less than nine are usually too small and boards of more than 20 are too large. With less than nine members, it becomes easy for a few individuals to have very loud voices, exercising more influence than might be healthy. With more than 20, it can be difficult to reach a consensus, keep all board members current, and make timely decisions in a turbulent environment. Sometimes too many cooks do indeed spoil the broth.

There are always exceptions. For example, one district hospital board in northern California has a five-member board and each member is on several committees, which seems to work for that hospital.

As a comparison, when the National Association of Corporate Directors (2001) completed a study on the optimum size of boards for public companies, almost 60 percent of the respondents said a board should be in the range of 8 to 11 members. For large companies (especially those found in the Standard & Poor's 500 index), boards tend to fall into the 9- to 12-seat range.

When evaluating their board's size, members should consider what needs to be done; what kind of expertise and skills would be useful; how current members cope with the workload required; and, if any of the above-identified pitfalls exist, essentially, how the current size really is working. Any changes in size can then be linked to the needs of the hospital rather than to personalities. In general, hospital boards in the 10- to 15-seat range seem to reach decisions and function more efficiently than do larger or smaller boards.

How Frequently Should a Board Meet?

...or, Is It Meeting Time Again?

Traditionally, healthcare boards almost always met monthly. Over the last ten years, an increasing number of boards have begun moving to quarterly or every other month schedules with the following results:

1. *Improved recruitment.* It is becoming more difficult to recruit and find good, experienced individuals to serve on boards. If potential board

members perceive your board as being efficient, effective, and utilizing time prudently, they are more likely to join you. If the image of the group is that it meets whether it needs to or not or spends time on trivial matters, the response will be less positive.

2. *More efficient utilization of time and information.* If a board goes from monthly to quarterly meetings, there is less time for extraneous matters and it will become essential for management to give the board governance information instead of management information. A board that meets quarterly is forced to utilize time efficiently. The board should insist on a biannual review of all the reports being given to it. Many board members will not say anything about receiving unnecessary information. They just won't read it and eventually may read nothing at all in advance of the meeting, affecting the board's efficiency and effectiveness. By reviewing the types of materials they are receiving, board members can indicate those they find inappropriate and focus solely on those of a governance nature. They will then be more inclined to read their materials, assured what they receive is indeed important to their purpose.

3. *More effective delegation to committees.* Much of a board's work is done in committees. Effective boards make sure that the right people chair their committees and that the right individuals are members of the committees. If the committees are structured and staffed with careful thought, their efforts will decrease the need for the board to duplicate the committee's work, and therefore the board can meet less frequently. Choosing the committee chairs is one of the most important jobs of the board chair.

It may be difficult to get a board to meet quarterly if it has been meeting monthly. However, it might move to meeting six times per year, and if that works, agree to move to quarterly meetings. True to human nature, boards tend to fill the amount of time allotted for a meeting, and if that time is reduced, members usually become aware of the need for more efficient meetings and look for ways to make this happen. Boards that have moved to quarterly meetings seem to spend time on governance rather than management activities, utilize their committees effectively, and have more success in recruiting new members.

What Basic Information Should Boards Receive for Board Meetings?

...or, Is All This Stuff Really Necessary?

It is important for boards to receive governance information rather than management information. All materials for discussion at a meeting should be sent to board members at least a week before any meeting. What should these different materials include?

1. *Minutes of the previous meeting.* The board should receive minutes from the previous meeting to give them a chance to read and refresh their memories about the discussions and the actions taken. Minutes should be brief but thorough and should reflect action taken, without a verbatim account of the discussion.

2. *Agenda for the coming meeting.* The CEO also should have been able to spend enough time with the board chair, who is responsible for the agenda, to develop a thoughtful and meaningful agenda addressing the key issues and reports in a logical sequence.

3. *Complete financial statements.* The board must receive complete financial statements at each meeting, along with dashboard financial indicators—the specific items the finance committee and board have agreed on that are particularly meaningful and that the board wishes to see in more detail at each meeting.

4. *A quality measurement report.* The board should always receive a quality measurement report that is meaningful and understandable. The report should contain quality indicators developed by the quality and community health committee and agreed to by the board, just as the financial indicators developed by the finance committee.

5. *Other reports and resource materials.* In addition to a progress report from the CEO and reports from its other board committees as appropriate to their work, the board should periodically receive materials regarding trends in healthcare. These resources should be educational and should help the board think strategically as it considers future options for the organization.

As previously noted, many boards receive entirely too much information, which members frequently do not bother to read. One giveaway is the member who arrives at a meeting with an obviously unopened packet of materials and who does not or cannot contribute to the discussion. Another is reports in materials packets that nobody seems to know much about and that are not discussed. When queried about why it received such a report, one board replied, "Bill insisted we get it and it just keeps coming." When asked why Bill wasn't at that particular meeting so he could be asked about it, the answer was, "Oh, Bill died four years ago."

To address these problems, the full board should review and evaluate the type of information it is receiving at least every two years to decide if it is appropriate and meeting members' needs. If not, changes should be made based on members' needs and suggestions.

What Criteria Should the Board Use in Selecting New Members?

...or, Who's a Likely Candidate?

The selection of new board members is one of the most important topics in this book. If members are identified and selected carefully, the subsequent work of the board should flow smoothly and creatively for the benefit of the organization. If members are selected with little thought other than "Gee, Judy's nice and has a great sense of humor," then the board would miss the opportunity to fill a talent void; run the risk of adding a difficult personality; or, worse still, bring on someone who is not actually interested in the organization at all.

Most district, county, and city boards do not have the luxury of making final selections, but even those boards can have some degree of influence. For example, district hospital board members run for election; therefore, current board members can actively look for individuals who meet at least some of the desired criteria and encourage those individuals to run. In county hospitals where county commissioners appoint board members, usually along political lines, the board can list criteria and encourage county commissioners to consider the criteria when appointing new board members. Recently, many district hospitals have begun converting to the 501(c)(3) status of private hospitals and, as such, will handle board appointments as discussed in the remainder of this section.

It can be very difficult for a hospital to compete and thrive in today's environment with the wrong people on the board. Some of Jim Collins's research in his book, *Good to Great*, relates directly to how important it is for boards of directors to select the right people for the board. Collins (2001) found in his research that the great companies

> ...first got the right people on the bus, the wrong people off the bus, and the right people in the right seats – and then they figured out where to drive it. The old adage that people are your most important asset turns out to be wrong; people are not your most important asset. The *right* people are.

Collins also found that in the great companies people clearly loved what they did, largely because they loved *whom* they did it with. I think the same is true with hospital boards; get the right people on the "board bus" (and the wrong people off) and the right people in the right seats, then figure out strategically where to go. The correct, carefully selected people on the bus will love what they are doing and with whom they are doing it.

Each board is likely to have some criteria that will be specific to that board. However, the following general criteria are extremely useful for overall consideration, and their use has resulted in the selection of some very good board members. This matching process is like pouring candidates into a funnel shaped by the criteria: only those who fit the criteria will fit through the funnel and begin to appear for selection. These criteria, in no particular order, are discussed below.

Experience

Find candidates who have some kind of board experience. The local chamber of commerce can be a useful source for those who are or have been on the boards of organizations in your area. The healthcare learning curve is quite steep for many individuals, so it is best to find those who already have a reasonable idea how to function in a board role—they won't have to learn two new roles simultaneously.

Achievement

Look for individuals who have accomplished something. It could be in building a business, serving on a board of an organization that provides a needed service to the community, doing something resulting in personal recognition, being an outstanding teacher in the high school or local college, or accomplishing anything that connotes personal achievement.

Occupation and skill

Boards go through stages where their attention needs to be focused on a specific portion of the organization's goals and objectives. Accordingly, different skill sets can be needed at different times. The board, or governance committee, should periodically determine what experience and skills would be useful and whether there are holes in the board's knowledge base that require filling.

Examples might include someone with in-depth financial skills or a quality care guru, or perhaps an individual who has worked with a construction or remodeling project would fill an empty niche. At times, the board may need to look outside the community for the missing expertise, but this is becoming more common for boards to do. The key is to find individuals who bring something to the table that will benefit the organization.

Team player

Being on a board is a team sport. People who do not play well with others in sandboxes are usually not good board members. Although exceptions exist, many times certain occupations have not provided team training. For example, sometimes entrepreneurs have difficulties because they are used to building businesses by themselves, being actively involved in several aspects of making the business grow, acting and not delegating, and in general wearing many hats at the same time. Often, surgeons—because of their training to make quick decisions, see instant results and be the "captain of the ship"—find being a team player difficult.

In a similar fashion, followers may also not make the best board members. These individuals frequently offer very little during a discussion, tending not to speak until everyone else has contributed and then ride in on the coattails of whoever they perceive is leading the group at that time. They bring nothing to the table, and the team derives no benefit from their presence.

Affluence

Affluence can be a controversial criterion, but one that should not be discounted. Affluent people have many times been very successful in business enterprises and know what it takes to get results. Affluent people often have a social conscience, plus the time to spend on a board. Affluent people can frequently better resist pressures from medical staffs, employee groups, community groups, or special interest stakeholder groups. This ability is particularly important in a smaller community where so many people know one other. Wealth alone should not disqualify anyone from board consideration.

Interest in and commitment to the organization

It is important to find board members who share an interest in and commitment to the organization's mission, values, goals, and objectives. The organization's mission and values should be reviewed with potential board members in enough detail to determine if the prospect really believes in them. Members of boards of children's hospitals throughout the United States almost always seem to have had a child treated at the hospital or a very close relationship with someone who had a child in the hospital. These individuals very clearly understand the hospital's mission, believe it, and are committed to it. Usually, if a children's hospital is having financial difficulties, the mission of taking care of sick children comes first, and how it is to be paid for comes second. Between effective fundraising, adherence to the mission, and strategic affiliations, children's hospitals seem to survive and some flourish. This is not to say that boards should adhere to activity that is leading the organization to a financial calamity. Rather, individuals on the board must know and support the hospital's mission to make sound decisions to advance the organization in a fiscally sound manner.

Personal qualities

Look for personal qualities that will make this individual a good board member. Does he have high integrity? Does she show compassion? Is he a good listener? Does she appear to have high morals? Is he intelligent? Will she make decisions based on facts and not emotion? These qualities will be very important, particularly if the organization faces difficult times when it must make hard decisions and speak with one voice.

Objectivity

This quality is crucial in a potential board member. Members serve on the board to function as a team for the benefit of the organization, its stakeholders, and the community it serves, not to advocate for social causes or represent a particular constituency such as a group of employees, special interest groups, or geographical areas. The board needs good members; whether they happen to be minorities, nurses, physicians, bankers, or trapeze artists should be of little consequence.

The only individual on the board who represents a constituency by virtue of his or her office is the president of the medical staff. This individual speaks for the medical staff and everyone else at the board table knows and expects it. They would, in fact, be surprised if he or she did otherwise.

Receptivity to training and evaluation

Look for board members who are receptive to training and self-evaluation. Someone who arrives on the board knowing it all frequently stalls the board's progress with preconceived ideas. The healthcare industry is complex; just because someone knows a particular industry does not mean that knowledge carries over to healthcare. Very specific knowledge sets pertain to components such as reimbursement, medical staff relationships, licensure of personnel, and quality measurements. The board must stay continually educated about such issues and the changes that affect the organization.

Board members must also be receptive to opportunities to do not only a board self-assessment process on a rather regular basis but to look objectively at what contributions they are making to the organization as individuals.

Willingness to devote the necessary time

The world's greatest board members are useless if they don't have the time to read their materials and attend meetings. If the board member does not have the time to devote to the organization, then all the other qualities are almost irrelevant. The hospital or healthcare system is in many instances the largest corporation in a community, having the most employees and the largest revenue base, and thus requiring the most talented board members available. But those members must have the time to contribute. A board cannot afford to have letterhead or ornamental directors.

In summary, trustees of all hospitals know being a board member today is much more difficult than it was even five years ago. Changes in reimbursement, the Balanced Budget Act, more and more medical treatments moving to an outpatient basis, shortages of essential personnel, and a much more polarized society make keeping hospitals solvent, particularly those in rural areas, a challenge. It is now more important than ever for the hospital to have a board that functions smoothly and comprises the best talent possible.

When the bus seats are filled with individuals possessing the characteristics outlined above, a board should be able to focus on creating the map of where the organization is going and how to get there instead of wasting time trying to figure out if there is any gas in the tank or what color the bus should be.

What Criteria Should the Board Use to Select a Board Chair?

... or, Who's in the Hot Seat This Time?

Next to selecting a CEO, the most important thing a board can do is elect the right person to be board chair. A good chair does not necessarily guarantee high levels of board effectiveness, but a bad one guarantees ineffective performance.

When making this determination, all board members must remember: the chair does not control the board; the board controls the chair. If the board allows the chair to control the direction and activities of the board, then every time a new chair is selected, the organization heads off in a different direction, losing stability and continuity.

Unlike board members, the chair should definitely have term limits. A board chair should not serve more than four years in that position. Being a board chair today requires energy and time; much longer than four years and many chairs will burn out and no longer be able to give their best to the position. Do not put your chair in a position to burn out.

Along with having term limits for the chair, the board should give serious consideration to adopting the chair-elect model. The board should have a system for determining who the next chair will be, a year before the present chair finishes his or her term. That gives the chair-elect a year to watch and learn from the present board chair and a year for the board to get used to who the next chair will be. This allows time for a smooth transition from one chair to the next.

The board should consider the following questions when electing a board chair (or chair elect):

1. Does this individual have the time and energy to devote to the position?
2. Will this individual be effective in providing a confidential sounding board for the CEO?

3. Does this individual demonstrate a good understanding of the organization and its long-term goals?
4. Does this individual understand the board's role as policymaker? Does he or she know the difference between governance and management?
5. Does this individual come to meetings prepared?
6. Does this individual make valuable contributions? Does he or she raise pertinent questions and provide valuable insights?
7. Is this individual respected by his or her board colleagues?
8. Is this individual a good listener who considers other's perspectives before making decisions?
9. Does this individual seem to understand the balance between discussing an issue fully and reaching decisions in a timely fashion?

Given the variables in human nature, some people who are very good board members may be very ineffective board chairs. There are those who are not comfortable in that kind of leadership position but who otherwise make invaluable contributions to the board's work. A smart board will not place someone in the role of chair if the individual does not wish to sit there. The position of chair is very important and the board should take the selection very seriously.

Who Are the Right Physicians for a Hospital Board?

...or, What's Up, Doc?

Although hospital boards should be working to ensure their membership includes a variety of talent who fits the identified needs of the organization, all boards usually have at least one physician on their rosters. As a group, physicians should know the hospital's primary business is caring for and treating sick people, and they should have an understanding of the reasons for a specific course of clinical action. "In addition to the president of the medical staff, we need the expertise of physicians on the board," says Patricia Bergin, president of the board of North Hawaii Community Hospital, Waimea, Hawaii. "However," Bergin adds, " they should think like board members first, with the hospital taking priority, and members of the medical staff second" (Biggs 2000).

President of the medical staff and other physician members

The president of the medical staff, by virtue of the position, is usually an ex officio member of the board. This individual basically serves one purpose and that is to represent the entire medical staff, a role that is generally understood by everyone involved. In this role, the medical staff president provides the board with input from an important group of stakeholders and can keep those stakeholders informed of board actions that affect their practices. No one expects the president of the medical staff to take any position on anything that is not favorable to the medical staff as a whole. "Everyone involved knows the role of the president of the medical staff, particularly the rest of the board, the administrator, and the medical staff itself. It is expected that the president of the medical staff will represent the view of the medical staff first," says Bergin (Biggs 2000).

The board should also determine if it needs participation from one or two other objective members who happen to be physicians. Unfortunately, whether an individual physician is the right one for the board at any given time can remain unknown until the individual is already in place. If a good selection process is in place, the uncertainty can be avoided. So how should these other physicians be selected?

Deciding which types of physicians are not eligible

Concern about conflict-of-interest issues appears to be at the top, or near the top, of most hospital boards' lists. Boards that participate in self-assessment programs are particularly interested in this topic; therefore, it is one to which boards who are selecting physician members should pay particular attention.

Although exceptions exist, the board nominating committee should eliminate all hospital-based physicians from consideration. This generally includes pathologists, radiologists, anesthesiologists, hospitalists, intensivists, medical directors, emergency room physicians, or any physician who is on the hospital's payroll or who has a contract with the hospital. Why?

As an example, it is very difficult for the hospital CEO to recommend a particular piece of expensive equipment not be purchased for radiology when the radiologist is a member of the board, or worse yet, is chairperson or an officer of the board. Likewise, when an anesthesiologist comes to the CEO and wants his or her group to have an "exclusive contract" with the hospital, but does not want the group to be prevented from providing anesthesia services to a competing surgery center, it can be problematic if the anesthesiologist is on the board. Further, when physicians who are on the hospital's payroll are also on the board, it is very difficult for the CEO to negotiate salary or salary increases, either "for the boss with the boss" or for himself or herself. These obvious conflicts of interest can be avoided if such physicians are not seated on the board in the first place.

Any one of the physicians mentioned above may also be put in a difficult position if other members of that physician's group put pressure on the physician because he or she is a member of the hospital board and colleagues pressure the physician to push their agenda items or proposals. "There may be other physicians who have a conflict of interest as the hospital develops strategies to deal with managed care organizations, particularly regarding capitated contracts," says Dan Coleman, president and CEO of the John C. Lincoln Health Network in Phoenix, Arizona. Coleman agrees "it is difficult to have physicians on the board who have any type of contract with the hospital" (Biggs 2000).

Deciding which types of physicians are eligible

The board nominating committee should next determine which types of physicians are least likely to have potential conflicts of interests. These categories would include those not employed by the hospital. Primary care physicians (family practitioners, internists, obstetricians, pediatricians, etc.) may be good candidates. Other candidates could include cardiologists, oncologists, infectious disease specialists, pulmonologists, general surgeons, orthopedic surgeons, and urologists.

> "In smaller communities, it is sometimes better to have primary care physicians, rather than specialists, on the board," says Doug McMillan, CEO, West Park Hospital, Cody, Wyoming. "Because of the politics involved, specialists on the board may participate in board decisions which are unpopular with primary care physicians. This can have a negative effect on patient referrals

to that specialist, and could ultimately affect the specialist's willingness to participate in tough decision-making activities of the board," adds McMillan (Biggs 2000).

"It is important to have primary care physicians on the board because much of their livelihood does not come from working in the hospital, and their decisions can be more objective," says Thaine Michie, vice chairman, Poudre Valley Health System, Fort Collins, Colorado (Biggs 2000).

It is also not a good idea to ask the medical staff for recommendations. They are represented at board meetings by their president, who is the main spokesperson for that group of stakeholders.

Selecting the physician candidate

The board, through its nominating committee, now should begin a methodical process of identifying specific physician candidates for the board. This methodical process should, of course, be similar to that utilized in selecting other board members. Essentially, the nominating committee should also use the same criteria for selecting physician board members as it uses for other members:

1. *Experience*. Physicians who have had no other board experience should not be selected. The hospital is too important to the community to serve as a learning ground for novices. The resumes of all members of the medical staff should be on file at the hospital and should be fairly current since all members of the medical staff have to be reappointed on a regular basis. Resumes of physicians who would not have a conflict of interest should be reviewed to ascertain if the physicians are on or have recently served on any other boards, whether they be corporations, churches, Boy Scouts, or other community-based groups.

    Physicians who have served on other boards should have a clear understanding of the importance of a board member's fiduciary responsibilities. "Physician board members need to understand what fiduciary responsibility really means. Above all else, the board has a fiduciary responsibility to act in the best interests of the hospital, not in the best interest of the physicians' personal practices or personal interests," says Dan Coleman (Biggs 2000).

2. *Achievement.* The resumes should also provide information about achievements of eligible physicians. Have they been elected to any offices by the local, state, or national medical society or by other groups on whose boards they have served? Have they received other types of awards from those groups or from their peers? Have they achieved something or been recognized for an activity outside of medicine? On what kinds of committees of the hospital have they served? Do they bring other knowledge or achievement experiences which would be of use to the board?

3. *Management skills.* Resumes may also be reviewed to determine if the physician has done anything to improve his or her management skills. What kind of continuing education programs has the physician attended in the last five years? Many physicians today are getting MBAs or attending short-term management courses sponsored by professional associations or universities. Is the physician the managing partner of his or her group practice? To maintain their present income levels in today's turbulent environment, physicians need creativity and skills in management, financial knowledge, and the management of people. These are skills that can be put to good use for the benefit of the hospital.

4. *Ability to be a team player.* Just as with other members, serving effectively on a board is not an individual sport. The board's nominating committee should look for indications that the physician is or can be a team player. Some clinical specialties tend to stress teamwork more than others, but most physicians are not trained to be team players. The hierarchical nature of the clinical training model does not prepare physicians to share decision-making authority with nonphysicians. Physicians are taught to look at a problem, review all the options, make a decision, and see if it was good or bad based on outcomes. All of this happens in a relatively short time frame. CEOs and boards make decisions and may not know for several years if the decision was good or bad. A physician who cannot adapt to this environment will quickly become frustrated and lose usefulness to the overall endeavor.

5. *Personal qualities.* Some personal qualities the nominating committee should consider include intelligence (which most physicians have),

compassion, willingness to be a good listener, and willingness to compromise. The physician must have high moral and ethical standards, and integrity is an absolute must.

6. *Objectivity*. Board members must also come to meetings with open minds and no personal agendas, willing to put the welfare of the institution first in all deliberations. Look for physician candidates who will be objective. No one board member should represent a specific constituency (except the president of the medical staff). This is difficult because professionals (such as physicians) tend to identify with peers and like-trained individuals, rather than with an organization. Most physicians who go through this type of hospital board selection process should be sensitive to the need to be objective. The use of job descriptions, which should be available for the board as a whole as well as for each board position, is helpful in maintaining board members' objectivity. Because of their training, physicians may relate to specific job descriptions better than other board members can.

7. *Receptivity to training and education*. Although physicians are also usually very receptive to continuing education and training, indications the physician candidate will be receptive to board education programs are important. While this is important for all board members, the physician's "rugged individualist" mentality noted above makes it doubly important for physician board members to be willing to continue learning about governance and issues that make for more effective governance.

Special considerations

In addition to concerns previously noted, boards of smaller hospitals in rural communities have a particularly difficult challenge because of the small number of physicians on the medical staff. If the hospital has nine physicians on the medical staff who live in the community and they belong to two different practice groups, it can be politically difficult to select one of them to be a board member (in addition to the president of the medical staff, who attends meetings because of his or her position). Selecting a physician from the same group as the medical staff president could leave the board open to charges of favoritism, while selecting a physician from the competing group might result in a lack of cooperation on certain issues. Such boards may wish to consider inviting a physician from another (noncompeting) community to sit on the board. Some hospital boards have successfully taken this approach with other positions. (See Bilchik 1999 and the section on selecting "outside directors" later in this chapter.)

> "Some hospital boards have added individuals from outside the hospital's service area, and the same can be done with a physician," says Hans Wiik, president and CEO, Health Future, Medford, Oregon. "The key is to find an outside physician who can challenge traditional thinking, add expertise and knowledge, and above all, be objective," adds Wiik (Biggs 2000). John McNeil, former CEO, North Hawaii Community Hospital, Waimea, Hawaii, also agrees that it may be a good idea for some hospitals to have physicians from outside the community on the board or to "find a recently retired physician who would be an objective board member" (Biggs 2000).

It is difficult for some hospitals to have physicians as board members. In district hospitals, for example, board members are elected by the community, so the only way to get good physician members on those boards is to convince the right physicians to run for election. Busy physicians may not be willing to do so. Public opinion not only will shape who is elected to the board, but grappling with public opinion versus meeting the hospital's needs may present challenges that do not appeal to the average physician.

County hospitals may have somewhat similar difficulties. Usually, the county commissioners appoint the hospital board of directors and they sometimes appoint board members along political lines. Historically, physicians have not been the most visible people in political circles, so they tend not to be appointed to these positions.

In these latter two instances, a board that desires physician input will have to evaluate its circumstances and essentially mount its own "political campaign" to either convince qualified physicians to run for elected office or to convince the county commissioners to appoint physicians with the needed expertise.

In summary, hospital boards must look at having one or two physicians as board members. Certain physicians, because of their relationship to the hospital, have more potential for a conflict of interest than do others. If the nominating committee of the board reviews potential physician candidates in a methodical manner and utilizes criteria such as experience, achievement, management skills, team playing ability, personal qualities, objectivity, and receptivity to training and education, they can enhance the board's ability to make good decisions for the smooth functioning of the board; the benefit of the community; and, most importantly, the quality of care available to the hospital's patients.

Should Boards Consider Individuals from Outside the Community as Members?

...or, Can Outsiders Come in?

Simply put, in today's turbulent environment, more healthcare boards are looking outside their communities for board members than ever before. While certainly not a major groundswell, it is something boards can consider when seeking new members. When a board determines that specific skills or experiences are needed but not really available in the community, it makes more sense to broaden the search area than to leave a need unfilled. "Outside" directors usually are independent and provide a different degree of objectivity than those living in the community. Someone from outside the hospital can constructively identify and challenge old board and management assumptions that may no longer be valid much more easily than someone closer to the situation.

In general, outside directors fall into the following three categories:

1. *Individuals with unique skills.* These individuals have unique skill sets such as risk management, familiarity with a market or region new to the organization, special financial skills, or skills in strategic planning or thinking. Many times these individuals will push local board members to think in a different way and prioritize differently. An example would be raising the importance of quality programs and measures to the same level as financial reports. In addition, outside reviewers such as financial ratings agencies definitely look at the quality of an organization's board

and management when issuing bonds. Having a few board members with special expertise and geographic reach can strengthen a rating agency's confidence in the organization.

2. *Physicians.* In some situations, the board feels it needs physician input beyond that provided by the president of the medical staff but is not comfortable adding another physician from the medical staff. The answer would be to recruit a physician from a nearby area. Care must be taken, however, to ensure the individual is not competitive with physicians on the medical staff or affiliated with a hospital in competition with the board's hospital.

   Some healthcare systems recruit physicians who have regional or national recognition in areas such as quality assurance. This could very well be a solution for many small communities. In a situation where there may be only six physicians in town, with three belonging to one group and three to another group, the board may feel more comfortable having a physician from outside the community on the board. Or, a community may have only four physicians, all practicing in one group. If that group decides to move procedures out of the hospital, considerable tension will ensue. In such an instance, it may be good to have a physician from outside the community on the board while the situation is resolved.

3. *Hospital CEOs.* Some boards and CEOs have found it very helpful to have another CEO from a different state or a noncompeting hospital on the board. These individuals can bring a lot of knowledge and objectivity to the board and help the board to understand many of the problems facing the average CEO. The outside CEO can also help the board put its own situation in perspective, by sharing how similar problems are handled in another location. Most boards and CEOs who have taken this approach seem very satisfied with it and supportive of the idea.

As noted, adding board members from outside the community is not a groundswell movement, but a sampling of organizations where the idea has been implemented includes Mobile Infirmary Medical Center, Mobile, Alabama; Oakwood Healthcare System, Dearborn, Michigan; Allina Health System, Minneapolis, Minnesota; Clarian Health Partners, Indianapolis, Indiana; Exempla Health, Denver, Colorado; and Intermountain Health Care, Salt Lake City, Utah.

Should Board Members Have Term Limits?

...or, Is It Time to Go Yet?

As most hospital board members know, being a board member today is a challenge. Nearly all hospitals operate in very competitive environments where reimbursement is constantly changing and where physicians fight to maintain their incomes, often in direct competition with the hospital. Many hospitals that function in this environment have term limits for board members, where individuals go off the board for at least a year after a set amount of time; subsequently, they may be nominated again for another term. Many governance authors recommend term limits as a method of ensuring turnover of board members. However, it is becoming more apparent that board term limits must be reexamined and hospitals that have them should review why.

Primary disadvantage of term limits

Hospitals are very complex organizations and, in many instances, the largest employer in a community. Service from knowledgeable and talented board members is required. However, in today's healthcare environment, it is becoming more difficult to recruit talented individuals to serve on hospital boards. And once recruited, no matter how talented they are, these individuals usually still need two to four years of education to understand the nuances of the healthcare industry as a whole and hospitals in particular. To lose such knowledgeable and experienced board members because of arbitrary term limits appears highly counterproductive.

Another approach

Rather than losing members in this fashion, it makes much more sense to periodically complete a board member performance appraisal and to not renominate board members who score badly in the process. "Term limits are a residual of the 1960s and 1970s when it was felt to be important that certain people be placed on nonprofit boards. A board appraisal process is a much more effective way to allow board members to resign or change their behavior than term limits," says Dr. Lee Seidel, a professor of health administration at the University of New Hampshire (Biggs 2001).

Parkview Episcopal Medical Center in Pueblo, Colorado, dealt with the issue of term limits in a very direct way. The hospital board had term limits for several years and found it was losing knowledgeable, experienced, and dedicated board members as a result. In 1993, the board voted to change the bylaws to eliminate term limits. "Being a good hospital trustee requires learning about a very complex industry and that takes time. We frequently found a trustee was becoming particularly effective just as we were losing that trustee because of term limits," says James Hadley, former chair of the Parkview board. "Also, with CEO turnover sometimes too high, it is important for the board to act as the organization's 'corporate memory' and for decisions to be made with a long term focus," says Hadley (Biggs 2001).

"There is no need to have term limits for board members as long as you have active and productive people. When the hospital goes through a board review process, members who are not productive may be asked to not stand for reelection," says Earl Bakken, chairman emeritus, North Hawaii Community Hospital, Waimea, Hawaii (Biggs 2001).

Annual selection

Inova Health System, a five-hospital system in northern Virginia, appointed a governance committee to research possible options for trustee selection. After reviewing most of the usual methods of selecting trustees, the board decided to elect board members annually, and to elect the chair for one five-year term. "The board felt this method was better than having term limits, and would keep the board members focused on how they were performing on a more regular basis," said Knox Singleton, president and CEO. "This method of selecting board members has worked very well for us and has helped members concentrate on their governance role and effective leadership for a large organization" (Biggs 2001).

The Washington, DC–based Health Care Advisory Board (1996) completed a study, "The Rising Tide," for its member organizations on appointing board members and has recommended trustees be elected on an annual basis. This enables the nominating committee to determine whether to renew individual trusteeships for another year. The role of the board chair and the nominating committee become extremely important in such a system, and these individuals need to be willing to make objective and sometimes difficult decisions. Performance appraisals can help.

Performance appraisals

To accomplish annual selection as smoothly and objectively as possible, a formal evaluation process should be set in place; ideally, the size of the board will be such that it does not become onerous and all consuming. This process will provide an opportunity to craft individual roles for each trustee, giving the trustee a clear sense of the purpose and importance of his or her role. Annual completion of the process will allow an opportunity to provide feedback to trustees on how they are perceived and how they can provide maximum benefit to the hospital. The process also paves the way for the board and a board member to part amicably when the member lacks certain skills or commitment.

The annual board member performance appraisal should be brief and of a manageable size and should be completed and reviewed with the board member by the chair of the board. There can be as few as five to ten questions, each of which is assigned points. The points are totaled, with a specified number of points deemed as satisfactory performance. Questions usually relate to a board member's attendance, meeting preparation, understanding of role, willingness to take appropriate risks, support of board decisions, knowledge of the healthcare industry, understanding results of decisions, dependability, ability to work with others, willingness to compromise, and so on. The use of performance appraisals allows the chair to monitor board composition over time, identify less effective trustees, and coach others to better performance. (See Appendixes 6 and 7 for sample evaluation forms for the chair to use in evaluating individual board members.)

The board member annual performance appraisal does not take the place of a periodic board self-assessment survey. The board self-assessment survey should contain questions about board performance and board perceptions. That survey is usually completed by board members and tabulated by an outside consultant, and is a major discussion item at a board retreat. (See the "What Is an Effective Board Self-Assessment Process?" section later in this chapter and Figure 6.1a for a sample survey.)

Chair of the board

Although the elimination of term limits for board members makes sense, there are reasons to limit the term as chair of the board to a fixed amount of time in office. "The board chair should change every two to four years. The learning curve is too much to learn in less than two years. The chair-elect model is a good one because it forces the board to focus on who should be the next chair and provides that person with at least a year to closely observe the role and responsibilities of the chair. A person may be a very good board member, but would not make a good chairperson, which the board needs to keep in mind when selecting a chairperson," says Dr. Lee Seidel (Biggs 2001). If a chair-elect model is used, the chair may wish to have that individual assist in the performance appraisal process.

"It is my experience that the board chair needs to have a high energy level. In today's hectic healthcare environment, most individuals have difficulty maintaining that level after three to five years as chair," says Dr. Richard Bogue, former director of governance programs at the American Hospital Association (Biggs 2001). Earl Bakken agrees, saying "the chairperson should change after a reasonable period as chair, say three to six years, before he/she loses interest or faces some burnout. However, the former chairperson should stay on the board" (Biggs 2001).

Summary

Hospital boards that have term limits may wish to consider changing their bylaws to eliminate them, implementing an annual selection and performance appraisal process instead. "Term limits alone will not be effective for any purpose. What the board really needs to concentrate on is development of specific criteria for selecting board members; development of an effective orientation and ongoing continuing education program for board members; implementing an effective performance appraisal process; and developing a succession program," says William Schirmer, former vice president, Quorum Health Resources (Biggs 2001). The board should also consider restricting the amount of time in the chair position to no more than five years.

Being a hospital trustee today is more difficult that it has ever been, and hospitals cannot afford to lose excellent trustees because of term limits, especially in this ever-changing environment.

Should There Be an Age Limit for Members of the Board?

...or, How Old Is Too Old?

Is there a time when someone can no longer make a positive contribution to a board's work? Certainly. But that time does not arrive at some arbitrarily established age. Just as with term limits, if there is an effective self-assessment process in place and the board chair evaluates each board member on a regular basis, age limits are not necessary. Extensive reviews of the scientific literature on aging, physical and mental abilities, and job performance lead to the conclusion that chronological age is not a good predictor of abilities or performance. McEvoy and Cascio (1989) reviewed 96 research studies spanning a 22-year period that examined the effect of age on performance and found performance did not decrease as age increased, as typically believed.

One 35-year study of intellectual development reported that age changes in cognitive functions occur slowly. For most people, declines in intellectual abilities are of a small magnitude until they reach their mid-70s (Schaie 1996). Older individuals may actually have higher motivation and job satisfaction than the young. In research that examined 185 studies, it was found that internal work motivation, overall job satisfaction, and job involvement were positively associated with age (Rhodes 1983).

It appears many of the declines formerly attributed to aging actually should be attributed to injury, illness, or lifestyle variables. Therefore, age averages are not good indicators of individual ability levels, and the average ability of a 60- or 70-year old is not a useful basis for estimating individual capabilities and limitations. Generally speaking, therefore, boards should not conclude that ability declines are so uniform, common, or dramatic as to warrant putting age limits on individual board members.

From another perspective, it can be very useful to have a few board members who have been around long enough to provide a "corporate memory" for the board. Clichés that reference needing to "learn from the past lest we repeat past mistakes" can often be painfully true. Understanding what has gone before can indeed help boards make better decisions; older, long-term members can be a bridge to that understanding.

Experience also is a great teacher, and board members, like all of us, learn from their personal experiences. Sometimes it takes considerable time to accumulate enough experience to be able to view the healthcare organization and its community as a total system and to make the right connections. Experienced individuals, in many instances, see problems and opportunities as a whole within a complete context, which then allows them to also see obvious solutions to many problems.

Dysfunctional board members can come in all shapes, sizes, and ages. Excellent board members are excellent because they come to meetings on time, read the distributed material before the meeting, act as team players, and support board decisions. Age is not the determining factor for success on a board; other attributes clearly seem to be the important components, and these will show up when the individual is evaluated. As a delightful example, one Midwestern board member is at least 86 years old, has been on his board for over 53 years, and is generally viewed as the best overall member of that board.

Because chronological age by itself is not an accurate indicator of ability or functional competence, other mechanisms for assessing a board member's ability to contribute should be utilized. A good self-assessment program and a process whereby the chair of the board can evaluate individual board members is much more effective than establishing age limits for board members. (See Appendixes 6 and 7 for sample evaluation forms).

Should Board Members Be Paid Director's Fees?

...or, Is This a Get-Rich-Quick Scheme?

Should members of nonprofit healthcare organizations' boards be paid director's fees? This is an issue that generates considerable debate, and for which there is likely no one-size-fits-all answer. Several authors have reviewed the pros and cons of compensating directors including: Alexander (1990), Pointer and Ewell (1994), Johnson and Johnson (1994), Witt (1987), Bowen (1994), Hadelman and Orlikoff (1999), and Hupfield (2000).

Some observations have shown healthcare boards who compensate their directors pay an amount that includes both a retainer and remuneration for each meeting attended. Although very few members may need the money, just knowing they are being compensated seems to raise their level of conscientiousness, particularly about attendance and meeting preparation. Other means of compensating directors include deferred compensation, healthcare benefits, life insurance, or other benefits. Officers and chairs of committees are sometimes paid an additional amount.

Few studies or surveys have been completed to assess how many healthcare organizations actually pay their directors, and little has been written about the results of those organizations that do. The few available studies (Clark Consulting 2003; Hoffman et al. 1989; Wyatt Company 1986) indicate somewhere between 12 and 25 percent of the hospitals (and systems) in the United States compensate their directors. Some anecdotal evidence indicates that healthcare organizations that compensate their boards have had a good experience recruiting new board members, have high attendance at board meetings, and have an easier time conducting self-assessment surveys.

It is strongly recommended that boards should at least consider paying director's fees. Generally, however, board members themselves will not bring up the subject, so it should be raised by the chairperson or the CEO. To help expedite such a discussion, the following summary includes the most common pros and cons about the issue.

Why directors should be paid

1. As previously noted, compensating board members, regardless of the amount paid, increases attendance and participation at meetings. Board members also appear to prepare better for meetings. Whatever their actual motivation, board members probably would not want to give the appearance of being paid for work they do not do. Members

who do not want to be compensated may donate the money back to the organization and even receive a tax deduction if they chose to do so.

2. Most chairs of compensated boards view compensation as a way to recognize board members' efforts, rather than as an incentive for better performance. Compensating a director sends a very clear message that the individual's work is important to a board whose work is important. The recognition that a board member's time is valuable, not only at board meetings but in preparation for those meetings, is given a concrete expression. The message also tells board members that the organization wants their full attention, and to achieve that, is willing to compensate.

3. Paying board members does not necessarily diminish the community-oriented and charitable mission of the hospital. Paying board members may allow participation by community representatives who might not otherwise be able to afford to serve, thus broadening representation on the board.

4. A growing number of CEOs report having trouble, especially in the last five years, recruiting qualified board members. Competition for good board members has increased in many communities, and the hospital may well be in a contest of sorts with organizations that already pay their board members.

5. Compensating board members allows more flexibility in recruitment. As previously discussed, a hospital may need to move outside its immediate community for desired expertise and such members can bring a different type of objective viewpoint to the job. However, it can be awkward to recruit such individuals if they are expected to pay their own travel and other expenses to participate in board activities.

6. Compensating directors of nonprofit healthcare organizations can help discourage the feeling that whatever they do or don't do is fine, since, after all, they are "only" volunteers.

Why directors should not be paid

1. One school of thought indicates the very essence of voluntary trusteeship precludes compensation—that is, volunteers get far greater satisfaction from their accomplishments, and they will make a greater

contribution because they function for purely altruistic reasons rather than monetary ones.

2. Board members may worry about the appearance of a conflict of interest if they receive payment for their services.

3. Compensating board members introduces an economic variable that may interfere with the board's ability to objectively conduct an honest and complete self-assessment program.

4. Some boards fear they could lose their indemnification privileges as volunteer directors if they are compensated because state laws are so vaguely written in this area. Most statutes make it clear that directors are expected to act in good faith within the scope of their official action and duties, but because they are so vague otherwise, any challenges will likely be decided by the courts.

5. There appears to be no scientifically based evidence that compensation improves recruitment or performance of trustees of nonprofit boards. As noted earlier, there is anecdotal indication that compensating directors improves attendance, but it has not been scientifically proven.

6. The relatively small amount many healthcare organizations could or would pay may not make much difference in attracting and retaining the most qualified individuals.

7. Although the amount that could/would be paid might be small, many directors feel the appearance of directors paying themselves sends the wrong message to the community about the board's concern for healthcare costs. In this era of mismanagement by companies, such as HealthSouth and Enron, this is not an image some boards want to risk having.

Finally, despite differing schools of thought, the issue of board member compensation deserves thorough review and discussion. Some organizations could very well consider board compensation as much of a financial investment in their future success as the compensation packages paid to the full-time executive management team. However, regardless of the outcome of such discussion, it can also be used as a lead-in for additional deliberations on topics such as the development of more effective leadership, why boards should complete a self-assessment survey, or commitment and motivation at the board level. More effective governance will increase the effectiveness of the organization.

What Is Included in an Effective Orientation Program for New Board Members?

...,or, What Are We Supposed to Do Now That We're Here?

Each healthcare organization is a unique entity, with its own structure and manner of functioning. Even the most experienced and knowledgeable new board member cannot be expected to arrive knowing those specific components. A well-planned orientation program will definitely help new board members learn their way around, understand their role, and greatly assist them in meeting both their own and the board's expectations.

When designing a meaningful orientation program, it is important to ask continuing board members what they know now that they wish they had known when they first joined the board. This information can then be included in the program's design as appropriate. Some continuing members may find such a program to be a welcomed refresher course for them; therefore, while they should not be discouraged from attending, they should not be allowed to dominate the sessions.

It can be difficult to cover everything that needs to be covered in one session. Between sessions, members will have time to think about what they have learned and to seek clarification about anything that is unclear at the next session. This type of planning has shown better overall retention and a higher level of members' satisfaction than trying to pack everything into one sitting.

The board chair and the CEO have very specific functions to perform in an orientation program; therefore, the following information should be covered:

1. *Job description.* The first priority at a new board member orientation is a review of the board member's job description (see Appendix 3). The chair needs to hand the new board member a copy of the job description to review together. It will be much more meaningful if this is done by the chair and not the CEO. New members can then start off understanding their place in the organization and can relate the rest of the orientation to that perspective. This is also an ideal time for the board chair to review the difference between governance and management information and how the board approaches dealing with its proper role.

2. *Conflict-of-interest policies.* Another portion of the orientation to be presented by the board chair is an explanation of the organization's conflict-of-interest policy and the conflict-of-interest disclosure statement. Again, this message will carry more weight coming from the board chair than the CEO. (Appendixes 1 and 2 provide samples of these materials.)

3. *Attendance and evaluation.* The final components for the board chair to cover should be expectations of attendance at board meetings and the evaluation processes. A copy of any evaluation forms being used (see Appendixes 6 and 7 for samples) should be shared and reviewed. Then, when both the board self-evaluation and the individual evaluations are performed, the new member will not be taken by surprise and will understand it is a normal part of the board's routine.

4. *Organizational structure.* Following the components presented by the board chair, the CEO should review the hospital's organizational structure with the new member. Key positions and their responsibilities should be discussed and the individuals who fill those positions, along with their backgrounds, should be identified. A simplified organizational chart is very helpful in understanding the actual structure of the organization.

5. *Review of the healthcare industry.* Many new board members will not be familiar with highlights of the healthcare industry and should be given this information by the CEO. It will be helpful for them to understand such things as where healthcare fits in the country's overall budget, how much that is per capita, and how that compares with other countries. Provide a look at statistics about the average U.S. hospital—including numbers of outpatient visits, surgical procedures, and emergency room visits—in comparison with your hospital's figures. It is always interesting to look at the number and types of hospitals; numbers of physicians, nurses, and other healthcare providers in the United States; and the number of people enrolled in managed care plans locally and across the country. Information about morbidity, mortality, and other quality measures is more readily available and will help to put your hospital's statistics into perspective. Attention should be given to the rapidly expanding field of complimentary and alternative medicine, including any local impact it has had. Also consider

providing new members with actual copies of the most recent health-care background information and educational materials that have been given to the rest of the board, so they will not be lost when such materials are discussed or used in meetings.

6. *Review of board manuals.* Material with which board members should be familiar and to which they will refer from time to time should be compiled and placed in a notebook that allows items to be added, deleted, or updated. The CEO should review this material with new members:

- Organization's bylaws
- Organization's mission, vision, goals, objectives, and strategic plan
- List of board members and resumes for each
- Overview of organization's market and main challenges
- Review of organization's competitors
- Characteristics of the most important stakeholder groups
- Review of organization's finances and quality measures
- Update on any specific projects with which the organization is involved or is contemplating involvement

Finally, the CEO should take the new board member on a tour of the hospital or, if a system is involved, on a tour of some of the main facilities within the system.

Throughout the orientation process, the new member should be made comfortable enough to ask questions and for clarifications and to request any additional information he or she deems useful. The goal is to acclimate the new board member to the board as quickly and smoothly as possible.

How Should the Board's Annual Retreat Be Structured?

...or, It Wasn't Raining When Noah Built the Ark

Whoever coined the saying "It wasn't raining when Noah built the ark" may well have been advising someone to schedule a board retreat before a crisis occurred. If the hospital board chair or CEO waits until a crisis does occur, it will probably be too late to accomplish much in that high-stress environment.

All boards should already be in the habit of having an annual retreat; if not, this lack should be remedied as soon as possible. Planning the annual board retreat is usually the responsibility of the governance committee or a special committee appointed by the chair, and the basic idea is to get the board members away, out of their home base, to a place where they can comfortably discuss, without distractions, key issues not normally covered during a regular board meeting.

A board retreat can provide an opportunity for planning, a chance to refocus on fundamentals, a vehicle for team building and strengthening trust and relationships among board members, and a venue to conduct the self-assessment of the board. It can also provide time to focus on potential problems before they actually become problems or on an opportunity before it is lost.

Several elements go into making a board retreat successful, including the following:

1. *Obtain obvious leadership support.* A board retreat will not be successful unless it is obvious the retreat is considered to be very important to the chair, CEO, and other officers of the board. The chair must make it clear the retreat is a priority and 100 percent attendance is expected.

2. *Get board input in the retreat planning process.* Board members are more likely to support the need for a retreat and participate actively if they have some input into the planning of it. Many planning committees find it helpful to send a brief questionnaire to the full board, asking about subjects to cover. The committee should accommodate all responses if possible, particularly if any particular patterns emerge.

3. *Schedule the event with ample notice.* If the chair expects to get 100 percent attendance at the retreat, it must be scheduled at least four to five months in advance. It also helps if the planning committee, in its preplanning questionnaire, has asked the board for input on the best time for the retreat—weekday or weekend—and for information about already scheduled plans that would preclude a member attending in any particular time frame. Every effort should be made to accommodate these responses and to plan the event around conflicts.

4. *Make it clear who is to attend the retreat.* If the board will be addressing very sensitive or confidential matters, then participation should be

limited to the board. If the purpose of the retreat is to look at future options for the organization and review certain types of data and presentations, then it is appropriate for key staff to attend. In general, most board members are reluctant to say what they really think about any controversial issues in front of nonboard members. Just be clear about what is to be accomplished and what issues are to be discussed.

5. *Select the right location.* The event should be a true retreat. The board needs to get away from where normal business is conducted. This does not have to be a great distance nor does it have to be exceedingly expensive, but board members must be far enough away from home so they won't be checking in with their staff regularly or leaving early to return to their offices. They need to be where they can comfortably get to know each other better and focus on the issues in detail, without distractions. Part of the duties of the committee planning the retreat is to explore different options for holding the retreat. Alternative meeting places may include country inns and resorts, campgrounds or lodges at state or national parks, spiritual retreat centers, university conference centers, and corporate retreat centers.

6. *Design the agenda carefully.* The best retreats tend to be built around a single, clearly defined theme. These retreats focus on one or two issues of importance to the board, and everyone understands the objectives. The agenda should not be too ambitious; better to have ample time to do good work on one issue than for the group to leave feeling frustrated because they could not deal with overly ambitious expectations. Make sure the issue or theme is not something that can be handled at a routine board meeting. At least half of the time should be allocated for the board members to fully discuss the issue(s). This is where the board members get to know each other and understand each other best. Most board members won't speak up if they feel rushed and that there is no time for their comments. Excellent outside speakers will not make up for the opportunity for board members to discuss an issue between themselves.

7. *Select the facilitator carefully.* Having the CEO or board chair facilitate the retreat will pretty much ensure a disastrous retreat. The CEO and/or the chair cannot participate fully as well as run the meeting, and it is unfair to ask them to try. Having the usual authority figure running

the meeting can also inhibit much discussion and will allow the retreat to fall into the pattern of a regular board meeting. Retaining the services of an experienced consultant to serve as a facilitator will keep the discussion moving forward, ensure everyone takes the opportunity to participate, and allow the CEO and chair to participate. An objective facilitator can more easily prevent the board from getting off track during discussions of difficult subjects and can make sure conclusions are reached in an appropriate time frame. The board chair or CEO can lead part of the discussion, depending on the issue, but a facilitator will make the retreat more successful and satisfactory for everyone.

8. *Plan adequate social time*. It is very important that the retreat schedule allows time for board members to get to know each other on a social basis. They will function better as a board and enjoy working together more if they come together as a team through social interaction. Even within small communities, all the board members do not necessarily travel in the same circles. Public boards, such as those involved with district or county hospitals, have a great need to become acquainted as individuals because they are not self-perpetuating and cannot decide who will be appointed by the county commissioners or elected by the public. Allowing adequate social time may very well be the most important part of a board retreat. If board members learn to know, respect, and get along with one other, they (just) might learn to govern better together.

9. *Develop an action plan for handling follow-up*. In general, boards take no votes and make no official decisions at a retreat. The retreat format should be designed to encourage full participation and creative thinking. Although conclusions should be reached so that no discussion is left hanging, formal votes should be left for subsequent business meetings.

   At the very least, the facilitator should be able to summarize the discussion in such a way that attendees can all agree with the result. That summary should ideally lead to development of an action plan with timetables so that the board agrees on what the next steps will be. It is a strange feeling to participate in a retreat, leave with one impression of what transpired, and then hear another's summary of the meeting—all of which makes you wonder if you were at the same meeting. The summary and action plan process can help prevent that disparity. The post-retreat interval can be used for staff or committees to tie up loose ends.

Summary

In summary, today's healthcare environment requires boards to function effectively and efficiently. In the past, boards were rather neutral entities who did not really help or hurt a hospital—the medical staff did its thing, administration did its thing, and the board had its annual fundraiser and everybody was relatively happy. Those days are gone—the board either helps or hurts the hospital now and there is no neutral ground. Boards must do everything possible to learn to work together, including retreats, continuing education, and learning as much as possible about the industry, all while still functioning at 30,000 feet. A board retreat is no longer considered the luxury it once might have been but has become an essential activity in which the board must engage. There should be a line item in the organization's budget for board education activities, including a retreat, to send the message to all that this is important to the board's work.

What Is an Effective Board Self-Assessment Process?

...or, Do We Have to Rate Ourselves?

Not too long ago, it was unheard of for boards to even think about the need to do a self-assessment, let alone to actually do one. However, as with so many other things in healthcare, that is changing, and recent upheavals in the corporate world almost compel any responsible board to take a closer look at how it functions. Boards that complete a self-assessment program seem to quickly solve many of their problems, even some that have plagued them for years. It is one more way for a board to fulfill its commitment to quality, for itself as well as for the hospital as a whole.

One example of a self-assessment process utilized by several hospitals is discussed here. Although there are many ways a board can complete the procedure, it is better to have an outside consultant coordinate the project than someone internal to the organization. This avoids any conflict of interest or appearance of conflict of interest, and board members seem to be more free to share their thoughts if an objective outsider is handling the survey tool and compiling the results. Steps in the process, regardless of who is coordinating, follow below.

Step One

Before a scheduled retreat where the board is going to do its self-evaluation, a survey tool is sent to board members for anonymous response. Figure 6.1a provides thirty sample questions that have been refined and updated on a regular basis. A deadline date for response return should be provided to encourage members to respond in a timely manner.

Step Two

The responses are sent to the consultant who tabulates the answers and identifies those areas where responses show a significant variance.

Interestingly, most boards appear to be in general agreement on 22 to 25 of the questions—that is, they strongly agree or agree and one or two members are in the somewhat disagree column. However, the responses on four to six of the questions will usually be all over the place, and on a rare occasion, the entire board will respond with disagree or strongly disagree on one of them. These are the questions the board needs to spend time addressing, and the consultant can help expedite that process.

In one example board's responses, there were four questions where board members had quite different answers. Using a shorthand version of the questions as given in Figure 6.1a, the differing responses to items 2, 13, 25, and 28 are shown in Figure 6.1b. There were 15 board members, and 15 response.

Figure 6.1a: Board of Directors Self-Assessment

Please check one answer for each question/statement. Results will be tabulated to reflect how board members feel about each question as a group. The questions are answered anonymously and no individual response is ever identified. The goal is to determine how the board as a group relates to these items.

Please return by ——————————————————————

Please fax your answers to ——————————————————————

1. Each board member is familiar with the hospital's current mission statement.
    ——strongly agree   ——agree   ——somewhat disagree   ——disagree
2. Proposals brought before the board are evaluated to ensure they are consistent with the hospital's mission.
    ——strongly agree   ——agree   ——somewhat disagree   ——disagree
3. The board has adopted a strategic plan, which is reviewed on a regular basis.
    ——strongly agree   ——agree   ——somewhat disagree   ——disagree
4. The board generally understands the concept of "co-option" whereby physicians cooperate with the hospital at times and compete with the hospital in other situations.
    ——strongly agree   ——agree   ——somewhat disagree   ——disagree
5. Participation of clinicians is sought in the governance process, to assist the board in fulfilling its responsibilities regarding the provision of quality patient care.
    ——strongly agree   ——agree   ——somewhat disagree   ——disagree
6. Membership on the board is open to physicians who function as regular board members (in addition to the president of the medical staff, who represents the medical staff).
    ——strongly agree   ——agree   ——somewhat disagree   ——disagree
7. The board reappoints individuals to the medical staff based on clearly established criteria and a medical staff recommendation.
    ——strongly agree   ——agree   ——somewhat disagree   ——disagree
8. The board reviews comparative statistical data on the quality of the hospital's clinical services and patient care and sets targets to ensure improvement.
    ——strongly agree   ——agree   ——somewhat disagree   ——disagree
9. The board reviews and adopts an annual budget, setting revenue and expense targets, and considers regular reports during the year to determine compliance.
    ——strongly agree   ——agree   ——somewhat disagree   ——disagree

10. The board approves specific parameters on items such as debt, liquidity, return on investment, and other financial ratios to provide early warning signals of financial problems.
    ———— strongly agree   ———— agree   ———— somewhat disagree   ———— disagree

11. The board adopts a long-term capital expenditure plan that estimates projected sources, costs, and uses of future funding for buildings and equipment.
    ———— strongly agree   ———— agree   ———— somewhat disagree   ———— disagree

12. Board policies and criteria for the selection of new members are clearly defined and followed to ensure continuing leadership and accessibility of needed knowledge and skills.
    ———— strongly agree   ———— agree   ———— somewhat disagree   ———— disagree

13. The board evaluates its performance to determine its effectiveness and to identify needed skills and knowledge for board continuity and growth.
    ———— strongly agree   ———— agree   ———— somewhat disagree   ———— disagree

14. The board periodically reviews its size, structure, committees, and tenure of members, officers, and committee chairpersons.
    ———— strongly agree   ———— agree   ———— somewhat disagree   ———— disagree

15. The board or its executive committee conducts an evaluation of the CEO each year using specific criteria agreed upon in advance with the CEO.
    ———— strongly agree   ———— agree   ———— somewhat disagree   ———— disagree

16. The board clearly understands the differences between the responsibilities of the board and management.
    ———— strongly agree   ———— agree   ———— somewhat disagree   ———— disagree

17. The board communicates effectively with the CEO regarding goals and expectations.
    ———— strongly agree   ———— agree   ———— somewhat disagree   ———— disagree

18. The board supports the CEO in his or her relationships with the medical staff.
    ———— strongly agree   ———— agree   ———— somewhat disagree   ———— disagree

19. The board has a policy regarding identification and resolution of real or perceived conflicts of interest by its members, physicians, and/or administrative staff.
    ———— strongly agree   ———— agree   ———— somewhat disagree   ———— disagree

20. All members of the board have job descriptions and understand their responsibilities, roles, and duties.
    ———— strongly agree   ———— agree   ———— somewhat disagree   ———— disagree

21. All members of the board participate in an orientation program and continuing education.
    ———— strongly agree   ———— agree   ———— somewhat disagree   ———— disagree

22. The board regularly reviews data about the medical staff to ensure future staffing will be adequate regarding numbers, specialties, and years in practice.

    —— strongly agree   —— agree   —— somewhat disagree   —— disagree

23. The chairperson ensures that all board members have equal opportunity to participate, time is not monopolized by a few, and agenda items are appropriately handled following adequate discussion.

    —— strongly agree   —— agree   —— somewhat disagree   —— disagree

24. The board has a written job description for the position of board chair.

    —— strongly agree   —— agree   —— somewhat disagree   —— disagree

25. The board has a clear chair selection and succession process, which is utilized.

    —— strongly agree   —— agree   —— somewhat disagree   —— disagree

26. The board has a position of chair-elect, or its equivalent, which is filled one year before the individual assumes the office of chair.

    —— strongly agree   —— agree   —— somewhat disagree   —— disagree

27. The chair's performance is evaluated by the board.

    —— strongly agree   —— agree   —— somewhat disagree   —— disagree

28. The board reviews and discusses emerging healthcare innovations and changes in medical technology as part of the continuing education programs that occur at each board meeting and during board retreats.

    —— strongly agree   —— agree   —— somewhat disagree   —— disagree

29. The board represents the hospital to the total community and does not advocate for any particular constituency or geographical area.

    —— strongly agree   —— agree   —— somewhat disagree   —— disagree

30. The members of the board generally utilize the services of the hospital for their own healthcare needs.

    —— strongly agree   —— agree   —— somewhat disagree   —— disagree

Comments: _____

_____

_____

_____

_____

_____

_____

_____

**Figure 6.1b: Example Summary of Responses
(Board of Directors Self-Assessment)**

Question	Strongly Agree	Agree	Somewhat Disagree	Disagree
2. Mission appropriate	3/15 (20%)	2/15 (13%)	6/15 (40%)	4/15 (26%)
13. Board performance	2/15 (13%)	6/15 (40%)	3/15 (20%)	4/15 (26%)
25. Chair selection process	4/15 (26%)	2/15 (13%)	5/15 (33%)	4/15 (26%)
28. Board reviews technology	4/15 (26%)	6/15 (40%)	2/15 (13%)	2/15 (20%)

Step Three

Following tabulation, the consultant assists the board in dealing with the results. The question is, how can the board most effectively discuss these four questions to see if changes can be made that will allow the board to more closely agree on them?

One technique that has produced some very good results is to divide the board into groups, with three to five board members per group. The four challenged statements from the survey—those having the most disagreement among board members—are rephrased into questions for each group to analyze.

For example, item 2 on the survey, "Proposals brought before the board are evaluated to ensure they are consistent with the hospital's mission," becomes Question One: "What can we as a board do to ensure that our decisions are consistent with our mission?" Item 13 on the survey, "The board evaluates its performance to determine its effectiveness and to identify needed skills and knowledge for board continuity and growth," becomes Question Two: "What can we as a board do to more effectively evaluate our own performance and the performance of each board member?"

Similarly, item 25 on the survey, "The board has a clear chair selection and succession process, which is utilized," turns into Question Three: "What do we need to do to improve our chair selection and succession process?" Finally, item 28, "The board reviews and discusses emerging healthcare innovations and changes in medical technology as part of the continuing education programs that occur at each board meeting and during board retreats," becomes Question Four: "How can we as a board improve our knowledge of new medical technology?"

Each group is then given a question to review, discuss, and to suggest solutions for. The suggested solutions are then put in an envelope and passed to the next group, which will repeat the process without looking at the prior group(s) suggestions. The questions continue around the groups in that fashion until they reach the last group that has not yet answered that question. This final group will review what the prior groups have suggested, add its own thoughts if they have not already been covered, and then craft a final recommendation for presentation to the entire board.

Using this technique, each board member has the opportunity to help identify problem areas and contribute to solutions; all board members become involved in creating viable solutions; and, before the retreat is over, the board has worked as a team to move forward in a positive fashion. When the work is done in this fashion, no one feels left out or personally challenged and a great precedent is set for handling any future challenges.

Acknowledgments

The "Who Are the Right Physicians for a Hospital Board?" section of this chapter is adapted and reprinted from *Trustee*, VOL. 53, NO. 9, by permission, October 2000. Copyright 2000, by Health Forum Inc. The "Should Board Members Have Term Limits?" section of this chapter is adapted and reprinted from *Trustee*, VOL. 54, NO. 2, by permission, February 2001. Copyright 2001, by Health Forum Inc.

References

Alexander, J. 1990. *The Changing Character of Hospital Governance*. Chicago: American Hospital Association.

Biggs, E. 2001. "Terminating Board Term Limits." *Trustee* (54) 2: 21–23.

———. 2000. "Selecting the Right Physician for Your Board." *Trustee* 53 (9): 22–23.

Bilchik, G. S. 1999. "Outside/In: Health Care Boards Look Beyond Their Communities for Trustees." *Trustee* 52 (7): 7–9.

Bowen, W. G. 1994. *Inside the Boardroom*. New York: Wiley.

Clark Consulting. 2003. "Healthcare Board of Directors Compensation Survey." Minneapolis, MN: Clark Consulting.

Collins, J. C. 2001. *Good to Great: Why Some Companies Make the Leap... and Others Don't*. New York: HarperCollins.

Hadelman, J., and J. Orlikoff. 1999. "Get Real. Professional Governing Boards Must Happen if Hospitals and Systems Are to Survive." *Modern Healthcare* 29 (41): 32.

Health Care Advisory Board. 1996. "The Rising Tide." Washington, DC: Health Care Advisory Board.

Hoffman, J. R., T. C. Hermann, D. R. Rich, R. L. Johnson, and S. L. Gill. 1989. "Compensation of Hospital Governing Boards: A National Survey." *Healthcare Executive* 4 (3): 34–35.

Hupfield, S. F. 2000. "Board Compensation: The Time Is Now." *Trustee* 53 (1): 28–30.

Johnson, E. A., and R. L. Johnson. 1994. *New Dynamics for Hospital Boards*. Chicago: Health Administration Press.

McEvoy, G., and W. Cascio. 1989. "Cumulative Evidence of the Relationship Between Employee Age and Job Performance." *Journal of Applied Psychology* 75 (1): 11–17.

National Association of Corporate Directors. 2001. 2001–2002 Public Company Governance Survey, 12–30. Washington, DC: NACD.

Pointer, D. D., and C. M. Ewell. 1994. *Really Governing: How Health Systems and Hospital Boards Can Make More of a Difference*. Albany, NY: Delmar.

Rhodes, S. 1983. "Age-Related Differences in Work Attitudes and Behavior: A Review and Conceptual Analysis." *Psychological Bulletin* 93 (2): 328–67.

Schaie, K. W. 1996. "Intellectual Development in Adulthood." In *Handbook of the Psychology of Aging*, edited by J. E. Birren and K. W. Schaie, 4th edition. San Diego, CA: Academic Press.

Witt, J. A. 1987. *Building a Better Hospital Board*. Chicago: Health Administration Press.

Wyatt Company. 1986. "Practices of Boards of Directors/Trustees in the Health Care Industry." Fort Lee, NJ: Executive Compensation Services.

CHAPTER SEVEN

Additional Information

How Should a Hospital Board Relate to Its Foundation?

...or, It's All in the Family

Foundation purpose and focus

Hospitals can raise money for themselves and their special projects in two different ways. Some hospitals place their fundraising activities in a separate hospital department and do not have a foundation at all. However, many hospitals have foundations separately organized to assume this responsibility. The foundation will have a board of directors that oversees the activities of the foundation and helps to raise funds.

Usually, when the hospital receives a larger-than-normal gift, the board considers forming a foundation and setting up a board of directors, following one of three available models:

1. A majority of foundation board members are hospital trustees
2. A minority of foundation board members are hospital trustees
3. The foundation board has only one or two hospital trustees and the hospital CEO as members

Most hospitals follow the third model, which is considered a truly independent foundation board, even though the hospital board or system board has the authority to approve appointments to the foundation board. Main reasons hospitals follow the independent foundation board model include the following:

- It reduces the possibility of "piercing the corporate veil," which means that if the hospital or related entity is sued, the plaintiffs cannot come after monies in the foundation because it is a separate corporation and does not have a majority or large number of trustees from the hospital board as members.
- Unless it chooses to do so, the hospital does not have to issue a consolidated financial statement. If foundation funds are shown in a consolidated statement, it will present an unrealistic view of both the hospital's actual financial status and that of the foundation. This skewed presentation could negatively affect donations to each entity.
- A foundation board separate from the hospital can focus exclusively on fundraising, leaving the hospital board to concentrate on hospital business.
- It is easier to separate out the actual costs of fundraising, allowing the hospital and foundation to know if they are efficiently raising money compared to other foundations.
- Many times, donors are more willing to donate money to a foundation that is separate from the hospital. The reasons for this may or may not be valid, such as having had a bad experience at the hospital and not wanting to support it. Some may also think the foundation is concentrating more specifically on investing and/or making better use of their donation.
- Because the work of the foundation board is quite different than that of the hospital board, the foundation board can be structured to represent more segments of the community, important for widespread community support in fundraising efforts.
- Some hospital trustees may not be comfortable as fundraisers. Being a trustee who is or should always be looking for possible donors is quite different than being a trustee for overseeing hospital operations.
- If hospital trustees are asked to serve on the foundation board, or vice versa, already busy people are being asked to become even busier.

- A final important reason for having separate boards is that foundation board service provides an excellent training ground for future hospital trustees.

Cooperation and support

It is very important the hospital board and the foundation board work closely together. The foundation board should never feel it is working hard to raise money for the hospital without being fully informed of hospital activities. To do so makes raising money for the hospital extremely difficult. The hospital board and administration are responsible for developing and maintaining cooperation between the foundation board and the hospital board.

The cooperation and support of the foundation board can be encouraged if the hospital board and administration do the following:

- Ensure foundation board members have a thorough orientation. They need to know the hospital's history, goals and objectives, and major challenges and have a description of their job as a foundation board member.
- Fully inform foundation board members about major decisions under consideration by the hospital board. It will be much easier to raise money if the foundation board understands why certain decisions are being made.
- Seek counsel from foundation board members as the hospital board gets closer to making a major decision. The foundation board may have a unique understanding of how donors or certain stakeholders will react to a particular decision.
- Always inform the foundation board of breaking news before telling the public. This will help the foundation board be supportive of the decision and provide an excellent sounding board for gauging public opinion.
- Establish an organized method for each board to report what it is doing to the other board. One simple way to do this is to have a regular item on each board's agenda for a report from the other.
- Include foundation board members when the hospital board is having board education sessions. Foundation board members need to have the

same level of knowledge about issues affecting the hospital as hospital board members do, and their understanding of these issues will strengthen their ability to speak on the hospital's behalf when raising funds.

- Involve the foundation board leaders, or the whole foundation board if appropriate, in the hospital's activities. Make sure they are invited to key social events or educational programs.
- Do everything possible to make foundation board members feel as if they are part of the hospital family.

Remember, an informed, involved, and motivated foundation board will be able to conduct its work in support of the hospital with enthusiasm. The familial relationship between foundation and hospital is one to be nurtured, for the satisfaction and benefit of both groups.

What Healthcare Jargon Would Be Helpful to Know?

...or, What Foreign Language Is This?

This little section is indeed little, but a book such as this would be greatly remiss if it did not comment on the "foreign" language of healthcare. As with many other industries, the healthcare arena has spawned its own lexicon, inhabited by a seemingly unending stream of abbreviations and special jargon that can be as confusing to board members as it is to the general public. CEOs of healthcare organizations, and others to whom the jargon is a normal part of their daily lives, must remember to communicate with their boards using as little healthcare terminology as possible because it can be intimidating, frustrating, and confusing for the listener.

As a personal example, I remember entering a doctoral program at a major university after being a hospital CEO and merging two hospitals. I was attending a general business faculty meeting and everyone kept referring to the problems they were having with the "OB" courses. I kept thinking to myself, "Why is obstetrics a problem here?" When I asked, I was told that in their setting "OB" referred to organizational behavior, not obstetrics.

Board members should never hesitate to ask what a term or concept means. They don't deal with the terminology on a daily basis and should not be expected to know the terms. Appendix 8 provides a basic list of common healthcare abbreviations and terms, which should be helpful as board members negotiate their way through this fascinating industry.

What Should the Board Know About Complementary and Alternative Medicine?

...or, Is This Snake Oil or Something Sound?

Complementary and alternative medicine (CAM) is defined as a group of diverse medical and healthcare systems, practices, and products that are not presently considered to be part of conventional medicine. For many CAM therapies, key questions are yet to be answered through well-designed scientific studies. Questions include ideas such as whether they are safe and whether they actually work for the diseases or medical conditions for which they are used. The list of those concepts considered to be CAM continually changes, as those modalities proven to be safe and effective—such as acupuncture, chiropractic, naturopathy, and massage therapy—become adopted into conventional healthcare and as new approaches to healthcare emerge.

Complementary medicine and alternative medicine differ from each other in one key way: complementary medicine is used with conventional medicine and alternative medicine is used in place of conventional medicine. An example of a complementary therapy is using aromatherapy to help lessen a patient's discomfort following surgery. An example of alternative medicine may involve the use of a special diet to treat cancer instead of using surgery, radiation, or chemotherapy as recommended by a conventional physician. To further complete the picture, "integrative medicine" is a term used to describe the combination of mainstream medical therapies and CAM therapies for which there is some high-quality scientific evidence of safety and effectiveness.

A growing number of U.S. hospitals are making CAM available to patients. According to Sita Ananth (2002), project director for CAM at the American Hospital Association (AHA), 15 percent of hospitals offer CAM therapies and 60 percent of medical schools offer courses in CAM. The following are findings from Ananth's 2002 AHA survey:

- A CAM service was twice as likely to be provided in an outpatient setting than in an inpatient one.
- Massage therapy, pastoral care, acupuncture, and biofeedback are the most popular outpatient services. Massage therapy, pastoral care, and relaxation treatment are the most frequent inpatient uses of CAM.
- Patient demand is the primary motivator for offering these services; other motivators are clinical effectiveness, the interest of new patients, and as a means of differentiating a hospital from its competitors.
- The primary challenges facing hospitals in implementing successful CAM programs include physician resistance, lack of budget, lack of internal expertise, and provider credentialing.
- One way to provide more CAM services while obtaining greater acceptance and reimbursement is to integrate them into existing programs.
- More than 70 percent of patients withhold information about their CAM use from their physicians. Physicians need to be trained to elicit this information from patients to be knowledgeable about their patient's total health status.
- Hospital administrators need to educate themselves about the credentialing of these providers and how it might fit within the hospital's structure. The most commonly used CAM therapies—acupuncture, chiropractic, naturopathy, and massage therapy—offer standardized national exams for their practitioners.

The National Center for Complementary and Alternative Medicine, a component of the National Institutes of Health, classifies the major types of CAM into five categories (NCCAM 2003):

1. *Alternative medical systems.* Alternative medical systems are built on complete systems of theory and practice. Often, these systems have evolved apart from and earlier than the conventional medical approach used in the United States. Examples of alternative medical systems developed in Western cultures include homeopathic medicine and naturopathic medicine. Examples of systems developed in non-Western cultures include traditional Chinese medicine, Ayurveda, and acupuncture.
2. *Mind-body interventions.* Mind-body medicine uses a variety of techniques designed to enhance the mind's capacity to affect bodily function and symptoms. Some techniques that were considered CAM in the

past have become mainstream (for example, patient support groups and cognitive-behavioral therapy). Other mind-body techniques are still considered CAM, including meditation, prayer, mental healing, and therapies that use creative outlets such as art, music, or dance.

3. *Biologically based therapies*. Biologically based therapies in CAM use substances found in nature, such as herbs, foods, and vitamins. Some examples include dietary supplements, herbal products, and the use of other so-called "natural" but as yet scientifically unproven therapies (for example, using shark cartilage to treat cancer).

4. *Manipulative and body-based methods*. Manipulative and body-based methods in CAM are based on manipulation and/or movement of one or more parts of the body. Some examples include chiropractic or osteopathic manipulation and massage therapy.

5. *Energy therapies*. Energy therapies involve the use of an energy field. One example is *biofield therapy*, which is intended to affect energy fields that purportedly surround and penetrate the human body. The existence of such fields has not yet been scientifically proven. Some forms of energy therapy manipulate biofields by applying pressure and/or manipulating the body by placing the hands in, or through, these fields. Examples include qi gong, Reiki (Japanese word representing universal life energy), and therapeutic touch.

The integration of CAM into existing programs and treatment in today's hospitals is growing. Board members need to be aware of this movement to determine if they wish their hospital to use CAM therapies or to what degree.

What Are the Best Web Sites for Board Governance Information?

...or, What's the Latest?

For the board member who has some time to learn about the healthcare industry, how boards should function, and best practices of governance, there are some good web sites to visit. Some of them are about organizations that require subscriptions to receive certain materials, but much of the information is free. The following web sites are worth reviewing:

1. *American Governance & Leadership Group*
   (www.americangovernance.com). The American Governance &
   Leadership Group (AG & LG) is a partnership of the American
   Hospital Association and James Orlikoff, Jerry Pogue, Dennis Pointer,
   and Mary Totten. AG & LG offers a subscription program for educational services and other consulting services.

2. *Board of Directors Network* (www.boarddirectorsnetwork.org). The
   Board of Directors Network is an Atlanta-based nonprofit research
   and advisory organization whose mission is to increase the number of
   women on boards. The organization works through awareness cam-
   paigns, meetings with corporate leaders, and annual reports providing
   data on public company boards.

3. *BoardSource* (www.boardsource.org). BoardSource, formerly the
   National Center for Nonprofit Boards, is a resource for practical information, tools and best practices, training, and leadership development
   for board members of nonprofit organizations worldwide. Through
   their educational programs and services, BoardSource works to help
   organizations fulfill their missions by building strong and effective
   nonprofit boards.

4. *The Business Roundtable* (www.brtable.org). The Business Roundtable is
   the association of chief executive officers of leading U.S. corporations
   with a combined workforce of more than 10 million employees in the
   United States. The Business Roundtable seeks to identify issues early,
   do its homework carefully, and try to understand the problems faced
   by government and business. Much research and work has focused on
   boards of directors, how they should be structured, and how they
   should function.

5. *The Chairman's Society* (www.chairmanssociety.org). The Chairman's
   Society is an organization exclusively for hospital board chairs and
   chairs-elect. Membership in the Society is by invitation only.
   Educational programs are predicated on the belief that chairs benefit
   from education in a collegial environment where they can learn not
   only from experts in the field but from others who have board chair
   experience.

6. *Conference Board* (www.conference-board.org). The Conference Board
   creates and disseminates knowledge about management, governance,

and the marketplace to help businesses strengthen their performance and better serve society. Working in the public interest as a global, independent membership organization, the Board conducts research, convenes conferences, makes forecasts, assesses trends, publishes information and analyses, and brings executives together to learn from one another.

7. *Corporate Directors Forum* (www.directorsforum.com). The Corporate Directors Forum is dedicated to promoting high standards of professionalism in corporate board directorship. They forge alliances among leadership in industry, academia, and government to generate corporate stakeholder values, while fostering high standards of ethics, diversity, and social responsibility. They also provide board-focused peer networking, "best practices" directorship education, governance advocacy leadership, director mentoring, and board recruitment resources.

8. *The Corporate Library* (www.thecorporatelibrary.net). The Corporate Library is intended to serve as a central repository for research, study, and critical thinking about the nature of the modern corporation, with a special focus on governance and the relationship between management and the board of directors. Most general content on the site is open to visitors at no cost; however, advanced research relating to specific companies and certain other advanced features are restricted to subscribers only.

9. *Encyclopedia About Corporate Governance* (www.encycogov.com). Encycogov is an academic encyclopedia about corporate governance intended for use by students, academics, business people, and government officials. The vision of Encycogov is to be the most useful and well-documented web-based resource about topics that are relevant for understanding issues in corporate governance. Encycogov was started in the summer of 1999 as an experiment and its development continues. The website is hosted by the Copenhagen Business School and the majority of Encycogov's visitors come from the United States and Great Britain.

10. *The Governance Institute* (www.governanceinstitute.com). The Governance Institute provides an education and development subscription service designed exclusively for health system and hospital

boards. Benefits include on-demand research services, access to the Institute's governance information clearinghouse, copies of research reports and white papers, copies of the bimonthly *Board Room Press* for all directors, and educational videos on key healthcare issues.

11. *Internet Nonprofit Center* (www.nonprofits.org). The Internet Nonprofit Center, which provides information for and about nonprofits, is a project of The Evergreen State Society based in Seattle, Washington. The Internet Nonprofit Center is the home of the Nonprofit FAQ. The FAQ is based on frequently asked questions— and their answers— drawn from the "Nonprofit" email discussion forum. There is much discussion about nonprofit organizations, the role of the board, the role of the CEO, and how to relate to volunteers.

12. *National Association of Corporate Directors* (www.nacdonline.org). Founded in 1977, the National Association of Corporate Directors (NACD) is an educational, publishing, and consulting organization focused on board leadership and a membership association for boards, directors, director-candidates, and board advisors. NACD promotes professional board standards, creates forums for peer interaction, enhances director effectiveness, asserts the policy interests of directors, conducts research, and educates boards and directors concerning traditional and cutting-edge issues. NACD is focused primarily on commercial corporations, but most of its services are useful to health system and hospital boards.

13. *Volunteer Trustees* (www.volunteertrustees.org). Volunteer Trustees is a national organization of nonprofit hospital and health system governing boards. The organization was founded in 1980 to give voice to the trustees of America's voluntary healthcare system and is dedicated to preserving and furthering the nonprofit healthcare sector. Volunteer Trustees provides a national forum run by trustees for trustee-to-trustee exchange, discussion, and education.

In addition to these web sites that focus primarily on the structure and functioning of boards, numerous other sites cover all aspects of healthcare, disease entities, healthcare statistics, and a myriad of other topics related to the healthcare industry. Happy surfing!

References

Ananth, S. 2002. "CAM: Complementary & Alternative Medicine." *Health Forum Journal* 45 (5): 47.

National Center for Complementary and Alternative Medicine. 2003. "What Is Complementary and Alternative Medicine (CAM)?" [Online article; retrieved 7/9/03.] www.nccam.nih.gov/health/whatiscam/.

EPILOGUE

As TRUSTEES OF all hospitals and healthcare systems know, being a board member today is much more difficult than it was even five years ago. With changes in reimbursement and the Balanced Budget Act and more medical treatments moving to an outpatient basis, just keeping a hospital solvent, particularly one in a rural area, is a challenge. One key to a healthcare organization's success is a board of directors that is composed of the best talent available and that functions smoothly with its CEO and within its community.

The increasingly turbulent business environment as a whole has caused increased focus on boards of directors in general, including those in healthcare. Just as boards in the public sector are receiving amplified scrutiny, communities and key stakeholders are watching to see if nonprofit boards are building long-term value and structuring themselves to make appropriate decisions and to see if they provide needed services to the community in an effective and efficient manner.

In the world of public, for-profit organizations, Jim Collins (2001) makes the point that boards have no responsibility to the group of people who buy and sell their stock with rapidity (shareflippers). Boards should instead concentrate on creating great companies that build value for the shareholders who hold their stock over the long term. Healthcare organizations could well approach their task with the same long-term thought in mind.

In this environment, healthcare boards need to consciously review their structure and assess how they function. This book has been designed to assist a hospital board in functioning effectively to achieving its goals. It can be used as a guide by new board members and for review by continuing members. Some boards will seek answers to some of the questions discussed here; others may utilize the questions and components in total. Some recommendations will fit certain hospitals more than others. Most recommendations, however, have universal application.

Boards that concentrate on structuring themselves for the long term will be more effective than their counterparts that do not. Boards with job descriptions, a defined selection process, a good orientation program, continuing education programs, a thorough self-assessment process, an understanding of their roles and responsibilities, and a continuing desire to relate to their key stakeholders and community will function smoothly for the benefit of their organizations.

Public company boards are coming under intense scrutiny recently with new requirements by the New York Stock Exchange, Securities Exchange Commission, NASDAQ, and the passage of the Sarbanes-Oxley Act of 2002. It is only a matter of time before many of these new requirements and regulations affect nonprofit healthcare boards. Many are already looking at what parts of these new regulations they should voluntarily begin implementing. For example, under the Sarbanes-Oxley Act, CEOs and CFOs must personally certify the accuracy of the organization's financial statements. Healthcare CEOs and CFOs in nonprofit organizations could do this now before it becomes a requirement.

The ideal governing board of a healthcare organization will be one that has looked at the types of information and recommendations in this book as a whole, decided which will improve that particular board's performance, and made the changes that fit. The modern healthcare board should strive to reach consensus and harmony with its community and key stakeholders. If just one key in this book helps unlock the door to accomplishing that, it is worthwhile. Good luck!

Reference

Collins, J. C. 2001. *Good to Great: Why Some Companies Make the Leap... and Others Don't*. New York: HarperCollins Publishers.

APPENDIX I

[Name of Organization]

Conflict of Interest Policy

Section 1. Purpose:

_____ is a nonprofit, tax exempt organization. Maintenance of its tax exemptions is important both for its continued financial stability and for public support. Therefore, the IRS as well as state regulatory and tax officials view the operations of _____ as a public trust, which is subject to scrutiny by and accountable to such governmental authorities as well as to members of the public.

Consequently, there exists between _____ and its board, officers, and management employees and the public a fiduciary duty, which carries with it a broad and unbending duty of loyalty and fidelity. The board, officers, and management employees have the responsibility of administering the affairs of _____ honestly and prudently, and of exercising their best care, skill, and judgment for the sole benefit of_____. Those persons shall exercise the utmost good faith in all transactions involved in their duties, and they shall not use their positions with _____ or knowledge gained therefrom for their personal benefit. The interests of the organization must be the first priority in all decisions and actions.

Section 2. Persons Concerned:

This statement is directed not only to directors and officers, but to all employees who can influence the actions of _____. For example, this would include all who make purchasing decisions, all persons who might be described as "management personnel," and anyone who has proprietary information concerning _____ .

Section 3. Areas in which Conflict May Arise:

Conflicts of interest may arise in the relations of directors, officers, and management employees with any of the following third parties:

1. Persons and firms supplying goods and services to _____ _____ .
2. Persons and firms from whom _____ leases property and equipment.
3. Persons and firms with whom _____ is dealing or planning to deal in connection with the gift, purchase or sale of real estate, securities, or other property.
4. Competing or affinity organizations.
5. Donors and others supporting _____ .
6. Agencies, organizations, and associations which affect the operations of _____ .
7. Family members, friends, and other employees.

Section 4. Nature of Conflicting Interest:

A conflicting interest may be defined as an interest, direct or indirect, with any persons or firms mentioned in Section 3. Such an interest might arise through:

1. Owning stock or holding debt or other proprietary interests in any third party dealing with _____ .
2. Holding office, serving on the board, participating in management, or being otherwise employed (or formerly employed) with any third party dealing with _____ .

3. Receiving remuneration for services with respect to individual transactions involving _____ .

4. Using _____ 's time, personnel, equipment, supplies, or good will for other than _____ approved activities, programs, and purposes.

5. Receiving personal gifts or loans from third parties dealing or competing with _____ . Receipt of any gift is disapproved except gifts of a value less than $50, which could not be refused without discourtesy. No personal gift of money should ever be accepted.

Section 5. Interpretation of this Statement of Policy:

The areas of conflicting interest listed in Section 3, and the relations in those areas which may give rise to conflict, as listed in Section 4, are not exhaustive. Conflicts might arise in other areas or through other relations. It is assumed that the directors, officers, and management employees will recognize such areas and relation by analogy.

The fact that one of the interests described in Section 4 exists does not necessarily mean that a conflict exists, or that the conflict, if it exists, is material enough to be of practical importance, or if material, that upon full disclosure of all relevant facts and circumstances it is necessarily adverse to the interests of _____ .

However, it is the policy of the board that the existence of any of the interests described in Section 4 shall be disclosed before any transaction is consummated. It shall be the continuing responsibility of the board, officers, and management employees to scrutinize their transactions and outside business interests and relationships for potential conflicts and to immediately make such disclosures.

Section 6. Disclosure of Policy and Procedure:

Transactions with parties with whom a conflicting interest exists may be undertaken only if all of the following are observed:

1. The conflicting interest is fully disclosed.

2. The person with the conflict of interest is excluded from the discussion and approval of such transaction.

3. A competitive bid or comparable valuation exists; and

4. The [board or a duly constituted committee thereof] has determined that the transaction is in the best interest of the organization.

Disclosure in the organization should be made to the chief executive officer (or if she or he is the one with the conflict, then to the board chair), who shall bring the matter to the attention of the [board or a duly constituted committee thereof]. Disclosure involving directors should be made to the board chair, (or if she or he is the one with the conflict, then to the board vice-chair) who shall bring these matters to the [board or a duly constituted committee thereof].

The [board or a duly constituted committee thereof] shall determine whether a conflict exists and in the case of an existing conflict, whether the contemplated transaction may be authorized as just, fair, and reasonable to _____ . The decision of the [board or a duly constituted committee thereof] on these matters will rest in their sole discretion, and their concern must be the welfare of _____ and the advancement of its purpose.

Source: Minnesota Attorney General's Office. 2002. "Suggested Non-Profit Organization Conflict of Interest Forms." St. Paul, MN: Attorney General of the State of Minnesota.

Note: The author would like to thank Gregory Piche, Health Law Division, Holland & Hart, Denver, Colorado, for his recommendations on this appendix.

APPENDIX 2

[Name of Organization]

Conflict of Interest Disclosure Statement

Preliminary note: In order to be more comprehensive, this statement of disclosure/questionnaire also requires you to provide information with respect to certain parties that are related to you. These persons are termed "affiliated persons" and include the following:

a. your spouse, domestic partner, child, mother, father, brother or sister;
b. any corporation or organization of which you are a board member, an officer, a partner, participate in management or are employed by, or are, directly or indirectly, a debt holder or a beneficial owner of any class of equity securities; and
c. any trust or other estate in which you have a substantial beneficial interest or as to which you serve as a trustee or in a similar capacity.

1. Name of Employee or Board Member: (Please print) _____

2. Capacity:

    _____ board of directors
    _____ executive committee

_____ officer

_____ committee member

_____ staff (position): _____

3. Have you or any of your affiliated persons provided services or property to _____ in the past year?   _____ YES   _____ NO

If yes, please describe the nature of the services or property and if an affiliated person is involved, the identity of the affiliated person, and your relationship with that person: _____

_____

_____

_____

4. Have you or any of your affiliated persons purchased services or property from _____ in the past year?   _____ YES   _____ NO

If yes, please describe the purchased services or property and if an affiliated person is involved, the identity of the affiliated person, and your relationship with that person: _____

_____

_____

_____

5. Please indicate whether you or any of your affiliated persons had any direct or indirect interest in any business transaction(s) in the past year to which _____ was or is a party?   _____ YES   _____ NO

If yes, describe the transaction(s) and if an affiliated person is involved, the identity of the affiliated person, and your relationship with that person:

_____

_____

_____

6. Were you or any of your affiliated persons indebted to pay money to _____ at any time in the past year (other than travel advances or the like)?   _____ YES   _____ NO

If yes, describe the transaction(s) and if an affiliated person is involved, the identity of the affiliated person, and your relationship with that person:

_____

_____

_____

7.   In the past year, did you or any of your affiliated persons receive, or become entitled to receive, directly or indirectly, any personal benefits from _____ or as a result of your relationship with _____, that in the aggregate could be valued in excess of $1,000, that were not or will not be compensation directly related to your duties to _____?
_____ YES _____ NO

If yes, please describe the benefit(s) and if an affiliated person is involved, the identity of the affiliated person, and your relationship with that person:

_____

_____

_____

8.   Are you or any of your affiliated persons a party to or have an interest in any pending legal proceedings involving _____?
_____YES _____ NO

If yes, please describe the proceeding(s) and if an affiliated person is involved, the identity of the affiliated person, and your relationship with that person: _____

_____

_____

9.   Are you aware of any other events, transactions, arrangements or other situations that have occurred or may occur in the future that you believe should be examined by _____'s [board of a duly constituted committee thereof] in accordance with the terms and intent of _____'s conflict of interest policy?   _____YES _____NO

If yes, please describe the situation(s) and if an affiliated person is involved, the identity of the affiliated person, and your relationship with that person:

_____

_____

_____

I HEREBY CONFIRM that I have read and understand _____'s conflict of interest policy and that my responses to the above questions are complete and correct to the best of my information and belief. I agree that if I become aware of any information that might indicate that this disclosure is inaccurate or that I have not complied with this policy, I will notify [designated officer or director] immediately.

_____   _____

Signature   Date

Source: Minnesota Attorney General's Office. 2002. "Suggested Non-Profit Organization Conflict of Interest Forms." St. Paul, MN: Attorney General of the State of Minnesota.

Note: The author would like to thank Gregory Piche, Health Law Division, Holland & Hart, Denver, Colorado, for his recommendations on this appendix.

APPENDIX 3

Board Job Descriptions

Chairperson of the Board

Function:

The Chairperson of the Board presides at all meetings of the board of directors and the executive committee, oversees implementation of corporate and local policies, ensures that appropriate administrative systems are established and maintained, while managing the actions and directions of the board.

The Chairperson of the Board represents the highest level of the board and works cooperatively with the organization's CEO.

Responsibilities:
- Directs the board and facilitates meetings
- Sets an example for other board members
- Ensures board members focus discussions on the common goals of the organization
- Serves as advisor to the CEO on matters of governance and board relations
- Serves as spokesperson of the organization for internal and external constituencies
- Serves as ex-officio member of all board committees, standing and ad hoc

- Designates chairs of board committees
- Delegates or executes the policies established by the board
- Calls special meetings of the board when necessary
- With the CEO, formulates board meeting agendas
- With the other officers and input from the board, monitors the performance of the CEO, including annual performance and salary reviews
- Aids in the recruitment and orientation of new board members
- Assumes other responsibilities and tasks as directed by the board

Vice-Chairperson of the Board

Function:
The Vice-Chairperson of the Board serves to fulfill the duties of the Chairperson in the event of his/her absence or disability and performs other duties as may be assigned by the Chairperson.

Relationship:
The Vice-Chairperson of the Board reports directly to the Chairperson.

Responsibilities:
- Performs the duties of the Chairperson in his/her absence
- Serves on the Executive Committee
- Chairs at least one major committee
- Assists the Chairperson in monitoring the implementation of board-established policies
- With the other officers and input from the board, monitors the performance of the CEO
- With the other officers and input from the board, conducts annual performance and salary reviews of the CEO
- Works closely with the Chairperson to develop and implement officer transition plans

Board Member

Function:
A board member serves to elect, monitor, appraise, advise, stimulate, support, reward, and when necessary or desirable, change top management.

Relationship:
A board member exists to meet the needs of the people the organization serves.

Responsibilities:
- Attends board meetings, arriving on time
- Reads agenda materials carefully prior to board meetings
- Participates in board orientation and continuing education
- Keeps all board deliberations confidential
- Avoids potential personal and/or professional conflicts of interest
- Approves annual budgets
- Understands the organization's mission and vision
- Avoids interference in hospital operations
- Establishes corporate policy
- Oversees physician recruitment and selection processes
- Develops and recommends strategic directions and financial plans for the organization
- Establishes evaluation criteria for key board officers and the CEO
- Elects officers (Chairperson, Vice-Chairperson, Treasurer, Secretary) at annual board meetings
- Represents the hospital to the community
- Participates in fundraising activities
- With the board officers, monitors the performance of the CEO
- Reviews results achieved by management in keeping with the organization's mission and goals

APPENDIX 4

Model Chief Executive Officer Employment Contract (Long Form)

This agreement, made and effective as of the day of _____ , 200X, between [name of Healthcare Organization], a corporation, and [name of CEO].

WHEREAS, the [Healthcare Organization] desires to secure the services of the CEO and the CEO desires to accept such employment.

NOW THEREFORE, in consideration of the mutual covenants contained in this Agreement, and intending to be legally bound, the [Healthcare Organization] and the CEO agree as follows:

1. The CEO will render fulltime services to the [Healthcare Organization] in the capacity of Chief Executive Officer of the corporation. The CEO will at all times, faithfully, industriously, and to the best of the CEO's ability, perform all duties that may be required of him by virtue of his position as Chief Executive Officer and all duties set forth in [Healthcare Organization] bylaws and in policy statements of the Board. It is understood that these duties shall be substantially the same as those of a chief executive officer of a business corporation. The CEO shall have and shall perform any special duties assigned or delegated to him by the Board.

2. In consideration for these services as Chief Executive Officer, the [Healthcare Organization] agrees to pay the CEO a base salary of $ ___

per annum or such higher figure as shall be agreed upon at an annual review of his compensation and performance by the Board. This annual review shall occur three months prior to the end of each year of the contract for the express purpose of considering increments. Salary shall be payable in accordance with the payroll policies of the [Healthcare Organization]. The CEO may elect to defer such portion of his salary to the extent permitted by law in accordance with policies established by the [Healthcare Organization].

3. (a) The CEO shall be entitled to _____ days of paid time off for vacation and sick leave each year, to be taken at times agreed upon by the Chairman of the Board.

   (b) In the event of a single period of prolonged inability to work due to the result of a sickness or an injury the CEO will be compensated at his full rate of pay for at least _____ months from the date of the sickness or injury.

   (c) In addition, the CEO will be permitted to be absent from the [Healthcare Organization] during working days to attend business and educational meetings and to attend to such outside duties in the healthcare field as have been agreed upon by the Chairman of the Board. Attendance at such approved meetings and accomplishment of approved professional duties shall be fully compensated service time and shall not be considered vacation time. The [Healthcare Organization] shall reimburse the CEO for all expenses incurred by the CEO incident to attendance at approved professional meetings, and such entertainment expenses incurred by the CEO in furtherance of the [Healthcare Organization's] interests, provided, however, that such reimbursement is approved by the Chairman of the Board.

   (d) In addition, the CEO shall be entitled to all other fringe benefits to which all other employees of the [Healthcare Organization] are entitled.

4. The [Healthcare Organization] agrees to pay dues to professional associations and societies and to such service organizations and clubs of which the CEO is a member, approved by the Chairman of the Board as being in the best interests of the [Healthcare Organization].

5. The [Healthcare Organization] also agrees to:
   (a) insure the CEO under its general liability insurance policy for all

acts done by him in good faith as Chief Executive Officer throughout the term of this contract;

(b) provide, throughout the term of this contract, a group life insurance policy for the CEO in an amount equivalent to $_____ ,
payable to the beneficiary of his choice;

(c) provide comprehensive health and major medical insurance for the
CEO and his family;

(d) purchase travel accident insurance covering the CEO in the sum of
$_____ ;

(e) furnish, for the use of the CEO, an automobile, leased or purchased
at the beginning of alternate fiscal years, and reimburse him for
expenses of its operation; and

(f) contribute on behalf of the CEO to a retirement plan qualified
under the Internal Revenue Code, at the rate of $_____ per
month.

6. The Board may, in its discretion, terminate this Agreement and the
CEO's duties hereunder. Such action shall require a majority vote of the
entire Board and become effective upon written notice to the CEO or
at such later time as may be specified in said notice. After such termination, the [Healthcare Organization] shall continue to pay the CEO's
then monthly base salary for the month in which his duties were terminated and for 24 consecutive months thereafter as an agreed upon severance payment. During this period, the CEO shall not be required to
perform any duties for the [Healthcare Organization] or come to the
[Healthcare Organization]. Neither shall the fact that the CEO seeks,
accepts, and undertakes other employment during this period affect
such payments. Also, for the period during which such payments are
being made, the [Healthcare Organization] agrees to keep the CEO's
group life, health, and major medical insurance coverage paid up and in
effect, and the CEO shall be entitled to outplacement services offered
by the [Healthcare Organization]. The severance arrangements
described in this paragraph will not be payable in the event that the
CEO's employment is terminated due to the fact that the CEO has been
charged with any felony criminal offense, or any misdemeanor criminal
offense related to substance abuse or to the operation of the
[Healthcare Organization], or has been excluded from Medicare,
Medicaid, or any other Federal Healthcare Program.

7. Should the Board in its discretion change the CEO's duties or authority so it can reasonably be found that the CEO is no longer performing as the Chief Executive Officer of the [Healthcare Organization] and/or its parent corporation, the CEO shall have the right, within 90 days of such event, in his complete discretion, to terminate this contract by written notice delivered to the Chairman of the Board. Upon such termination, the CEO shall be entitled to the severance payment described in Paragraph 6, in accordance with the same terms of that Paragraph.

8. If the [Healthcare Organization] is merged, sold, or closed, the CEO may, at the CEO's discretion, terminate this Agreement or be retained as President of the [Healthcare Organization], any successor corporation to or holding company of the [Healthcare Organization]. If the CEO elects to terminate his employment at such time, he shall be entitled to the same severance arrangement as would be applicable under Paragraph 6 if the [Healthcare Organization] had terminated his employment at such time. Any election to terminate employment under this Paragraph must be made prior to the [Healthcare Organization's] merger, sale, or closure, as applicable. If the CEO elects to continue to be employed by the [Healthcare Organization] or its successor organization, all of the terms and conditions of this Agreement shall remain in effect. The [Healthcare Organization] agrees that neither it nor its present or any future holding company shall enter into any agreement that would negate or contradict the provisions of this Agreement.

9. Should the CEO in his discretion elect to terminate this contract for any other reason than as stated in Paragraph 7 or 8, he shall give the Board 90 days written notice of his decision to terminate. At the end of the 90 days, all rights, duties, and obligations of both parties to the contract shall cease and the CEO will not be entitled to severance benefits.

10. If an event described in Paragraph 6, 7, or 8 occurs and the CEO accepts any of the severance benefits or payments described therein, the CEO shall to the extent not prohibited by law be deemed to voluntarily release and forever discharge the [Healthcare Organization] and its officers, directors, employees, agents, and related corporations and their successors and assigns, both individually and collectively and in

their official capacities (hereinafter referred to collectively as "Releasees"), from any and all liability arising out of employment and/or the cessation of said employment. Nothing cointained in this paragraph shall prevent the CEO from bringing an action to enforce the terms of this Agreement.

11. The CEO shall maintain confidentiality with respect to information that he receives in the course of his employment and not disclose any such information. The CEO shall not, either during the term of employment or thereafter, use or permit the use of any information of, or relating to the [Healthcare Organization] in connection with any activity or business and shall not divulge such information to any person, firm, or corporation whatsoever, except as may be necessary in the performance of his duties hereunder or as may be required by law or legal process.

12. During the term of this employment and during the 24-month period following termination of his employment, the CEO shall not directly own, manage, operate, join, control, or participate in or be connected with, as an officer, employee, partner, stockholder, or otherwise, any other hospital, medical clinic, integrated delivery system, health maintenance organization, or related business, partnership, firm, or corporation (all of which hereinafter are referred to as "entity") that is at the time engaged principally or significantly in a business that is, directly or indirectly, at the time in competition with the business of the [Healthcare Organization] within the service area of the [Healthcare Organization]. The service area is defined as [describe by counties, zip codes, a mileage radius, etc.]. Nothing herein shall prohibit the CEO from acquiring or holding any issue of stock or securities of any entity that has any securities listed on a national securities exchange or quoted in a daily listing of over-the-counter market securities, provided that at any one time the CEO and members of the CEO's immediate family do not own more than 1 percent of any voting securities of any such entity. This covenant shall be construed as an agreement independent of any other provision of this Agreement, and the existence of any claim or cause of action, whether predicated on this Agreement or otherwise, shall not constitute a defense to the enforcement by the [Healthcare Organization] of this covenant. In the event of actual or threatened breach by the CEO of this provision, the

[Healthcare Organization] shall be entitled to an injunction restraining the CEO from violation or further violation of the terms thereof.

13. The CEO shall not directly or indirectly through his own efforts, or otherwise, during the term of this Agreement, and for a period of 24 months thereafter, employ, solicit to employ, or otherwise contract with, or in any way retain the services of any employee or former employee of the [Healthcare Organization], if such individual has provided professional or support services to the [Healthcare Organization] at any time during this Agreement without the express written consent of the [Healthcare Organization]. The CEO will not interfere with the relationship of the [Healthcare Organization] and any of its employees and the CEO will not attempt to divert from the [Healthcare Organization] any business in which the [Healthcare Organization] has been actively engaged during his employment.

14. Terms of a new contract shall be completed, or the decision not to negotiate a new contract made, not later than the end of the tenth month. This contract and all its terms and conditions shall continue in effect until terminated.

15. This contract constitutes the entire agreement between the parties and contains all the agreements between them with respect to the subject matter hereof. It also supersedes any and all other agreements or contracts, either oral or written, between the parties with respect to the subject matter hereof.

16. Except as otherwise specifically provided, the terms and conditions of this contract may be amended at any time by mutual agreement of the parties, provided that before any amendment shall be valid or effective it shall have been reduced to writing and signed by the Chairman of the Board and the CEO.

17. The invalidity or unenforceability of any particular provision of this contract shall not affect its other provisions, and this contract shall be construed in all respects as if such invalid or unenforceable provision had been omitted.

18. This agreement shall be binding upon the [Healthcare Organization], its successors and assigns, including, without limitation, any corporation into which the [Healthcare Organization] may be merged or by

which it may be acquired, and shall inure to the benefit of the CEO, his administrators, executors, legatees, heirs, and assigns.

19. This agreement shall be construed and enforced under and in accordance with the laws of the State of _____ .

20. Any controversy, dispute, or disagreement arising out of or relating to this Agreement, or the breach thereof, shall be settled by arbitration, which shall be conducted in _____ , in accordance with the American Health Lawyers Association Alternative Dispute Resolution Service Rules of Procedure for Arbitration, and judgment on the award rendered by the arbitrator may be entered in any court having jurisdiction thereof.

This contract signed this day of _____ , 200X.

[NAME OF HEALTHCARE ORGANIZATION]

WITNESS:_____   BY:_____

(Board Chair)

WITNESS:_____   BY:_____

(Name of CEO)

Annotations to Chief Executive Officer Model Contract

This contract is the long-form CEO contract. It is somewhat more formal than the letter of agreement and specifically lays out some of the minimal benefits that a CEO should receive. Its formality and extensiveness make it more applicable as part of the negotiations for a new relationship than as a contract proposed during an existing one. It should be examined so that the items covered are raised in the negotiations rather than for the exact benefit and salary structure stated. Some benefits will be agreed upon and some not. That is the purpose of a contract negotiation.

Paragraph 1

This paragraph sets forth the duties of the Chief Executive Officer in very general terms. The specific duties of the CEO are not spelled out in the contract itself for two reasons. First, since the CEO should be involved in virtually every area of hospital operations, he/she must not be hamstrung by a limited "laundry list" of duties that narrowly circumscribe the scope of his/her responsibilities. Such lists relegate the CEO to the status of a "hired hand." In addition, since the duties of the CEO constantly change as the hospital changes, it is unwise to lock him/her and the hospital into a set routine from the start. The contract likens the CEO's role to that of a CEO in a business corporation to underscore the broad responsibility entrusted him/her.

Paragraph 2

This paragraph contains the financial terms of the contract, specifically, the CEO's salary. An annual figure is inserted in the first blank, while a monthly pay rate should be included in the second blank. The latter, of course, can be a weekly or bimonthly rate, depending on how the hospital or executive payroll is structured. After each annual salary review, the CEO's salary will presumably increase. New salary levels should be contained in a letter to the CEO from the Board Chairman, which will become incorporated into the initial contract. By the contract language, the CEO is also permitted the discretion to direct that a portion of his salary go into tax shelters as deferred income to the extent permitted by law.

Paragraph 3

This paragraph deals in general with compensation for time spent by the CEO away from the hospital, including vacation, sick leave, and out-of-hospital business. An alternative to laying these benefits out in the contract is to include them in a separate letter agreement.

Subparagraph 3(a) deals with vacation time for the CEO. Vacation time is compensated at the CEO's full rate and can be accumulated over the life of the contract.

Subparagraph 3(b) deals with sick leave in a similar fashion except that, unlike vacation time, it cannot be accumulated.

Subparagraph 3(c) deals with disability payments in the event of a major sickness or injury to the CEO. It can take the place of or supplement any disability insurance policy that the CEO may have in effect.

Subparagraph 3(d) permits the CEO to attend professional or hospital association meetings. The meetings to be attended should be agreed to in advance, or expense accounts should be approved after the fact by the Chairman of the Board. According to this clause, the CEO is entitled to reimbursement for all expenses and for full salary while in attendance at these meetings. Also, the travel expenses of the CEO's spouse and any necessary business entertainment expenses are also paid for. It should be stressed that the Chairman of the Board should approve all expense accounts of the CEO, for the CEO's own protection.

Paragraph 4

The CEO's dues for professional associations, service organizations, or clubs are paid for by the [Healthcare Organization], so long as his/her membership in them is reasonably related to the interests of the [Healthcare Organization]. It should not be necessary that these be approved in advance, but the Chairman of the Board should approve the organizations joined by the CEO.

Paragraph 5

Subparagraph 5(a) requires the [Healthcare Organization] to include the CEO under its general liability insurance policy for coverage for any acts done in good faith during the course of his/her duties. This is absolutely essential since CEOs are often named in lawsuits by patients alleging negligence or by physicians alleging improper denial or termination of medical staff appointment. The [Healthcare Organization] must protect the CEO if he/she is to carry out his duties innovatively, aggressively, and effectively.

The fringe benefit described in **subparagraph 5(b)** provides the CEO with a group life insurance policy, paid for by the [Healthcare Organization]. Of course, the CEO may name the beneficiaries of this policy.

Subparagraphs 5(c) and **(d)** respectively provide for comprehensive health insurance and travel accident insurance paid for by the [Healthcare Organization]. The health insurance package may be with Blue Cross/Blue Shield, a commercial carrier, or the [Healthcare Organization's] own self-insurance mechanism.

Subparagraph 5(e) provides for an automobile to be used by the CEO, the expenses of which are to be borne by the [Healthcare Organization].

Finally, **subparagraph 5(f)** permits payments into a retirement plan, which are over and above the CEO's base salary.

Paragraph 6

This clause is commonly referred to as the termination provision. It is by far the most important part of the contract. In the event that a majority of the Board members decide that the services of the CEO are no longer required, for whatever reason, the contract is terminated. However, the CEO will still be entitled to a stated amount of salary even though he/she is no longer working for the [Healthcare Organization]. Also, the CEO's group life and health insurance benefits continue. Outplacement services are also made available.

The exact number of months of severance pay to which the CEO is entitled is, of course, the subject of negotiation. The figure determined upon should accurately reflect the risks and challenges of the position.

This provision relieves the [Healthcare Organization] from its obligation to pay the severance arrangements in the event that the CEO's employment is terminated due to being charged with a criminal offense.

The purpose of this clause is to protect the CEO from threats of termination aimed at making him/her act with unnecessary caution. It is in the interest of the Board, the [Healthcare Organization], and the patients. The CEO must be able to exercise authority to the fullest extent possible. He/she must also be able to make hard decisions without fear that the job may be in jeopardy simply because someone on the Board or the medical staff did not like his/her choices.

Paragraph 7

This paragraph is similar to Paragraph 6, except that it comes into play in the event that the Board substantially changes the duties of the CEO, either by appointing another officer with similar duties or restricting the authority of the existing CEO. This would be one way to avoid the applicability of the severance provisions of Paragraph 6. As in the case of Paragraph 6, the CEO will be entitled to full salary for two years after termination plus group life and health insurance benefits.

Paragraph 8

This paragraph provides for severance payments in the event of merger or closure of the [Healthcare Organization].

Paragraph 9

This clause allows the CEO to voluntarily terminate the employment relationship, but if he/she does, no severance payment is made.

Paragraph 10

This paragraph protects the [Healthcare Organization] from needless future litigation by the CEO if the CEO accepts the severance benefits. This allows the [Healthcare Organization] to conduct its business relationship with the CEO without unnecessary caution. It is in the interest of the Board, the [Healthcare Organization], and the patients. This waiver will be enforced to the maximum extent allowable by law.

Paragraph 11

This provision protects the [Healthcare Organization] from disclosure of confidential information by the CEO during and after his/her term of employment with the [Healthcare Organization]. An employment contract with a key executive should contain a provision that prohibits the employee from disclosing to outsiders confidential information acquired by the employee during the term of employment without the express written permission of the employer. This provision should describe the applicable information so as to put the employee on notice as to what constitutes confidential information.

Paragraph 12

An employment contract with an executive employee typically contains a covenant by the employee not to compete with the employer during the term of the contract and for a specified period of time following termination of employment. The covenant is essential to the employer to prevent the employee from dealing with the employer's customers or otherwise engaging in competitive activities with the employer immediately following termination of employment so as to cause material adverse financial consequences to the business of the employer.

Restrictive employment covenants have generally been held to be valid where the restraint imposed on the employee is no greater than necessary to protect the legitimate business interests of the employer, and where neither the hardship to the employee nor the likely injury to the public outweighs the employer's need for protection. Thus, a covenant not to compete is usually upheld if it is clearly and reasonably limited as to time and area, and does not extend beyond the duration and geographical scope necessary for the protection of the employer. It should be noted that such restrictive covenants are unenforceable in some states.

Paragraph 13

This provision prevents the CEO whose employment at the [Healthcare Organization] has been terminated for whatever reason from recruiting other key executives to leave the hospital and join independent ventures excluding the [Healthcare Organization's] involvement.

Paragraph 14

This paragraph makes it simple for the [Healthcare Organization] and the CEO to continue the agreement beyond its initial term by signing a simple letter of agreement as an extension. The letter need only state that the initial contract has been extended for another specified period and set out the CEO's new salary. All of the initial provisions and benefits continue in force during the extension.

Paragraph 15

This is a standard clause that appears in most contracts. It states that this particular contract embodies total agreement of the parties and supersedes any previous contract, in response to the so called "parole evidence rule" of contract law. It eliminates any questions there may be as to the subject matter contained in the contract.

Paragraph 16

This provision requires that any amendments to the contract have to be stated in writing. This prevents either side from claiming that an oral understanding superseded some portion of this contract. It is technically referred to as a "no oral modification" or "NOM" clause.

Paragraph 17

This is known as a "savings clause." In the event that any portion of the contract is declared invalid or unenforceable by a court, the rest of the contract still remains in effect. The contract can therefore not be terminated on a technicality.

Paragraph 18

This paragraph keeps the contract in force even though the [Healthcare Organization] may change its corporate structure or be sold to another owner. It also provides that any benefits provided under the contract, such as life or accident insurance, that survive the CEO upon death, inure to the benefit of his/her estate or heirs.

Paragraph 19

This clause stipulates what law applies to the contract. This is especially useful in healthcare organizations near state lines. The law governing the contract should always be that of the state in which the [Healthcare Organization] is located.

Signatures

The execution of the contract should be authorized by the Board. It should be signed by the Chairman of the Board and the CEO, and should be witnessed by two individuals who are not on the Board and who are not members of the CEO's family. It should be filed along with other essential corporate documents. A copy should be given to the CEO. Needless to say, the terms of the contract, especially those relating to salary levels, fringe benefits, and termination, should be treated as confidential.

Source: American College of Healthcare Executives. 2003. "Model CEO Emplyment Contract." Chicago: ACHE.

APPENDIX 5

Sample Multirater CEO Performance Appraisal Instrument

This is an example of a partial multirater CEO performance appraisal instrument. It is not complete in that it does not include all of the questions normally asked on a CEO evaluation. Most appraisals use the computer to process the evaluation, so the rater would receive an electronic file. Using the computer allows great flexibility and almost any criteria can be evaluated, such as how well the CEO or the board follows the mission statement.

Performance feedback for (Name of CEO) _____

CEO for (Name of Organization) _____

Name of Respondent: _____

Position of Respondent: _____

Return completed form NO LATER THAN: _____

Please read instructions carefully before completing this questionnaire.

Instructions

Thank you for participating in the feedback process. Your time and effort are appreciated. Please give careful thought to your feedback in order to identify strengths and provide a basis for improvement. Do not rate higher or lower than deserved.

Your feedback is confidential. Your name will never be linked to the feedback you give. Other people will also contribute feedback. Your ratings will be combined (without your name) with their ratings to produce an average score, which will be summarized in a feedback report. No one can see your feedback without your password.

When writing comments, describe both positive and constructive aspects. The best comments are very specific and include examples. Avoid emotional comments, whether positive or constructive. You may change your feedback at any time, even after exiting the program. Simply click on the person's name, then click "Next" to review or change your feedback.

Questions

How satisfied are you with the performance of (Name of CEO) _____ ?

CEO for (Name of Organization) _____

1. Involves the medical staff, management staff, and employees as appropriate in planning strategy for growth of clinical services into the future.

1	2	3	4	5	6	7	8	9	10	N/A
Not satisfied		Minimally satisfied		Moderately satisfied		Very satisfied		Totally satisfied		

Constructive feedback: *What, if any, improvements are desired?* Please describe specifically. _____

_____

_____

_____

2. Maintains trust by listening effectively and communicating accurately on important issues affecting medical staff, management staff, and employees.

1	2	3	4	5	6	7	8	9	10	N/A
Not satisfied		Minimally satisfied		Moderately satisfied		Very satisfied		Totally satisfied		

Constructive feedback: *What, if any, improvements are desired?* Please describe specifically. _____

_____

_____

_____

3. Is visible within the hospital and available to the medical staff and hospital personnel.

1	2	3	4	5	6	7	8	9	10	N/A
Not satisfied		Minimally satisfied		Moderately satisfied		Very satisfied		Totally satisfied		

Constructive feedback: *What, if any, improvements are desired?* Please describe specifically. _____

_____

_____

_____

4. Conveys an understanding of the business of healthcare delivery.

1	2	3	4	5	6	7	8	9	10	N/A
Not satisfied		Minimally satisfied		Moderately satisfied		Very satisfied		Totally satisfied		

Constructive feedback: *What, if any, improvements are desired?* Please describe specifically. _____

_____

_____

_____

5. Provides leadership that engenders feeling of loyalty by medical staff and hospital personnel.

1	2	3	4	5	6	7	8	9	10	N/A
Not satisfied		Minimally satisfied		Moderately satisfied		Very satisfied		Totally satisfied		

Constructive feedback: *What, if any, improvements are desired?* Please describe specifically. _____

_____

_____

_____

6. Demonstrates a value system that shows dedication to the community based on customer satisfaction, mutual respect, integrity, and creativity.

1	2	3	4	5	6	7	8	9	10	N/A
Not satisfied		Minimally satisfied		Moderately satisfied		Very satisfied		Totally satisfied		

Constructive feedback: *What, if any improvements are desired?* Please describe specifically. _____

_____

_____

_____

7. Builds an effective management team with the consent of the Board.

1	2	3	4	5	6	7	8	9	10	N/A
Not satisfied		Minimally satisfied		Moderately satisfied		Very satisfied		Totally satisfied		

Constructive feedback: *What, if any improvements are desired?* Please describe specifically. _____

_____

_____

_____

8. Supervises all business affairs and ensures that all funds are collected and expended to the best possible advantage.

1	2	3	4	5	6	7	8	9	10	N/A
Not satisfied		Minimally satisfied		Moderately satisfied		Very satisfied		Totally satisfied		

Constructive feedback: *What, if any improvements are desired?* Please describe specifically. _____

_____

_____

_____

9. What else would you like to communicate to (Name of CEO) _____ ?

_____

_____

_____

10. What is (Name of CEO) ————————————'s most outstanding asset?

_____

_____

_____

_____

11. Add any final comments that you think would be helpful in improving this multirater performance appraisal instrument.

_____

_____

_____

_____

Source: Tyler, J. L., and E. L. Biggs. 2001. *Practical Governance*. Chicago: Health Administration Press.

APPENDIX 6

[Name of Organization]

Board Member Annual Performance Appraisal
(Short Version)

	Exceeds Expectation	Meets Expectation	Below Expectation
A. Board member is current in knowledge and understanding of the following:			
1. Goals and mission	____	____	____
2. Regionwide priorities	____	____	____
3. Hospital's financial status	____	____	____
4. Quality of care issues	____	____	____
B. Board member has been able to devote sufficient time to board responsibility, including reviewing and analyzing board materials before each meeting.	____	____	____
C. Board member has participated actively and knowledgeably during board meetings.	____	____	____
D. Board member's skill set is relevant to current competitive environment.	____	____	____
E. Board member has satisfactory working relationships with the board chairman, other board members, and CEO.	____	____	____

_____   _____
Board Member   Date

_____   _____
Chairman   Date

APPENDIX 7

[Name of Organization]

Board Member Annual Performance Appraisal (Long Version)

	Limited (1)	Acceptable (2)	Expected (3)	Impressive (4)	Exemplary (5)
1. Commitment:					
a. Prepares for meetings	___	___	___	___	___
b. Holds hospital interest as high priority	___	___	___	___	___
c. Reads, and participates in board education programs	___	___	___	___	___
2. Understands role:					
a. Knows appropriate organizational channels of operation	___	___	___	___	___
b. Considers other view-points	___	___	___	___	___
c. Willing to compromise	___	___	___	___	___
3. Decision making:					
a. Strives for necessary information	___	___	___	___	___
b. Willing to make decisions with less than total information when necessary					
c. Takes appropriate risks	___	___	___	___	___

	Limited (1)	Acceptable (2)	Expected (3)	Impressive (4)	Exemplary (5)
d. Supports board decisions	___	___	___	___	___
e. Challenges decisions, with cause	___	___	___	___	___
4. Analytical skills:					
a. States issues and problems clearly and concisely	___	___	___	___	___
b. Conclusions reflect good judgment and thoughtful evaluation	___	___	___	___	___
c. Understands results of decisions	___	___	___	___	___
d. Opinions and comments reflect adequate knowledge of healthcare industry	___	___	___	___	___
5. Dependability:					
a. Follows through on commitments	___	___	___	___	___
b. Reports and projects are on time	___	___	___	___	___
6. Personal traits:					
a. Remains poised under stress	___	___	___	___	___
b. Tactful	___	___	___	___	___
c. Appropriate appearance	___	___	___	___	___
d. Gets along with people	___	___	___	___	___
e. Sensitive to other's feelings	___	___	___	___	___
Total each column	___	___	___	___	___

GRAND TOTAL: _____

———— 22-24 Limited
———— 45-66 Acceptable
———— 67-88 Expected
———— 89-110 Impressive

Action Taken: ————————————————————————————————
——
——
——
——
——
——
——
——
——

Director	Date
Chairman	Date

APPENDIX 8

Common Healthcare Abbreviations and Terms

AAHP   American Association of Health Plans
AAPCC   average adjusted per capita cost
ACHE   American College of Healthcare Executives
ADS   alternative delivery systems

AHA   American Hospital Association or American Heart Association
AIDS   acquired immune deficiency syndrome
ALOS   average length of stay
AMA   against medical advice *or* American Medical Association

ANA   American Nurses Association
ANP   advanced nurse practitioner
ART   accredited record technician
ASC   ambulatory surgery center

BBA   Balanced Budget Act of 1997
BBRA   Balanced Budget Relief Act of 1999

BMR	basal metabolism rate
BP	blood pressure
CAH	critical access hospital
CAM	complementary and alternative medicine
CAT	computerized axial tomography
CBC	complete blood count
CCU	cardiac care unit
CDC	Centers for Disease Control
CMI	case mix index
CMS	Centers for Medicare & Medicaid Services
CNM	certified nurse midwife
CNS	central nervous system
CON	certificate of need
CPR	cardiopulmonary resuscitation
CQI	continuous quality improvement
CRNA	certified registered nurse anesthetist
CVA	cerebrovascular accident, a stroke
CVI	cerebrovascular insufficiency
D&C	dilatation and curettage
DC	Doctor of Chiropractic
DDS	Doctor of Dental Surgery
DME	durable medical equipment
DNR	do not resuscitate *or* do not report
DO	Doctor of Osteopathy (osteopathic physician)
DPM	Doctor of Podiatric Medicine
DRG	diagnosis related group
DVM	Doctor of Veterinary Medicine
ECF	extended care facility
EEG	electroencephalogram

EENT	eye, ear, nose, and throat
EKG, **ECG**	electrocardiogram
EMG	electromyogram
EMS	emergency medical services
EMT	emergency medical technician
ENT	ear, nose, and throat
FFS	fee-for-service
FI	fiscal intermediary
FQHC	federally qualified health center
FTE	full-time equivalent
GI	gastrointestinal
GP	general practitioner
GU	genitourinary
HHS	U. S. Department of Health and Human Services (federal)
IPA	independent practice association
IVA	intravenous
JCAHO	Joint Commission on Accreditation of Healthcare Organizations
LOS	length of stay
LTC	long-term care
MCO	managed care organization
MD	Medical Doctor (allopathic physician)
MOB	medical office building
MRI	magnetic resonance imaging
MSA	metropolitan statistical area
MSO	management service organization
ND	Doctor of Naturopathic Medicine or Nursing Doctorate

OB-GYN	obstetrics and gynecology
OD	Doctor of Optometry
OSHA	Occupational Safety and Health Administration
PCN	primary care network
PET	positron emission tomography
PHO	physician hospital organization
POS	point of service
PPO	preferred provider organization
PPS	prospective payment system
PSA	prostate specific antigen
PSO	provider sponsored organization
QA	quality assurance
QI	quality improvement
RBC	red blood count
RBRVS	resource-based relative value scale
SARS	severe acute respiratory syndrome
SIDS	sudden infant death syndrome
SNF	skilled nursing facility
SPECT	single photon emission computerized tomography
Stark I & II	physician referral laws—part of OBRA 1989 (Stark I) and 1993 (Stark II)
Stat.	immediately
T&A	tonsillectomy and adenoidectomy
TB	tuberculosis
Temp.	temperature
TQI	total quality improvement
TQM	total quality management
UR	utilization review
WBC	white blood count

Acuity. A term used to describe the degree or severity of illness.

Acquired Immune Deficiency Syndrome (AIDS). A fatal, incurable disease caused by a virus that can destroy the body's ability to fight off illness, resulting in recurrent opportunistic infections or secondary diseases afflicting multiple body systems.

Acute Care Hospital. Typically a community hospital that has services designed to meet the needs of patients who require short-term care for a period of less than 30 days.

Advance Directive. Written instructions recognized under law relating to the provision of healthcare when an individual is incapacitated. An advance directive takes two forms: living wills and durable power of attorney for healthcare.

Adverse Selection. The tendency of people who are in poorer-than-average health to apply for insurance coverage.

Allowable Expenses. The necessary, customary, and reasonable expenses that an insurer will cover.

Allowed Charge. Term used by Medicare to define the amount of a bill it will consider for payment.

Alternative Delivery Systems. Health services provided in other than an inpatient, acute care hospital, such as skilled and nursing facilities, hospice programs, and home health care.

Ambulatory Care. Medical care provided on an outpatient basis.

Ambulatory Payment Classification (APC). The method CMS uses to classify outpatient services and procedures that are comparable clinically and in terms of resource use. Serves as the basis of the Medicare outpatient PPS.

Ancillary. A term used to describe services that relate to a patient's care such as lab work, x-ray, and anesthesia.

Average Adjusted Per Capita Cost (AAPCC). The methodology used to develop the premium rate paid to HMOs by the federal government for Medicare recipients in a given geographic region based on historical service costs.

Average Daily Census (ADC). The average number of hospital inpatients per day. The ADC is calculated by dividing the total number of patient days during a given period by the number of calendar days in that period.

Average Length of Stay (ALOS). The average number of days in a given time period that each patient remains in the hospital. ALOS varies by type of admission, age, and sex. To calculate ALOS, divide the total number of bed days by the number of discharges for a specified period.

Benchmarking. A process that identifies best practices and performance standards to create normative or comparative standards (benchmark) as a measurement tool. By comparing an organization against a national or regional benchmark, providers are able to establish measurable goals as part of the strategic planning and total quality management (TQM) processes.

Board Certified. Describes a physician who is certified as a specialist in his or her area of practice. To achieve board certification, a physician must meet specific standards of knowledge and clinical skills within a specific field or specialty. Usually, this means completion of a supervised program of certified clinical residency and the physician passing both an oral and written examination given by a medical specialty group.

Board Eligible. Describes a physician who has graduated from a board-approved medical school, completed an accredited training program, practiced for a specified length of time, and is eligible to take a specialty board examination within a specific amount of time.

Brain Death. Total irreversible cessation of cerebral function as well as the spontaneous function of the respiratory and the circulatory systems.

Capital Expense. An expenditure that benefits more than one accounting period such as the cost to acquire long-term assets. Capital investment decisions typically involve large sums of money for long periods of time and have a major impact on the future services provided by an organization.

Capitalize. To record an expenditure that may benefit a future period as an asset rather than as an expense of the period of its occurrence (e.g., research and development costs).

Capitation. Method of payment for health services in which the insurer pays providers a fixed amount for each person served, regardless of the type and number of services used.

Cardiac Catheterization. A procedure used to diagnose disorders of the heart, lungs, and great vessels.

Case Management. A managed care technique in which a patient with a serious medical condition is assigned to an individual who arranges for cost-effective treatment, often outside a hospital.

Census. The number of inpatients who receive hospital care each day, excluding newborns.

Centers for Medicare & Medicaid Services (CMS). The federal agency responsible for administering Medicare, Medicaid, and the State Children's Health Insurance Program. CMS is formerly the Health Care Financing Administration.

Chemotherapy. In the treatment of disease, this is the application of chemical reagents that have a specific and toxic effect on the disease-causing microorganism.

Closed Panel. A managed care plan that contracts with or employs physicians on an exclusive basis for services and that does not allow those physicians to see patients from other managed care organizations. Staff model HMOs are examples of closed-panel managed care plans.

Code Blue. Indicates an emergency situation has occurred and mobilizes staff to respond.

Community Rating. A method of calculating health insurance premiums in which the health status and plan use of employer groups and individuals are combined and a single rate is paid by all groups and individuals.

Computerized Axial Tomography (CAT). Diagnostic equipment that produces cross-sectional images of the head and/or body.

Concurrent Review. A managed care technique in which a representative of a managed care firm continually reviews the charts of hospitalized patients to determine if they are staying too long and if the course of treatment is appropriate.

Consolidated Omnibus Budget Reconciliation Act (COBRA). Federal law that requires employers with more than 20 employees to extend group health insurance coverage for at least 18 months after employees leave their jobs. Employees must pay 100 percent of the premium.

Consumer Price Index, Medical Care Component. An inflationary measure encompassing the cost of all purchased healthcare services.

Cost Shifting. A phenomenon in which providers are inadequately reimbursed for their costs by some payers and subsequently raise their prices to other payers in an effort to recoup costs. Low reimbursement rates from government healthcare programs often cause providers to raise prices for medical care to private insurance carriers.

Credentialing and Privileging. Process by which hospitals determine the scope of practice of practitioners providing services in the hospital; criteria for granting privileges or credentialing are determined by the hospital and include individual character, competence, training, experience, and judgment.

Critical Access Hospital (CAH). Part of the Medicare Rural Hospital Flexibility Program created by Balanced Budget Act of 1997. A critical access hospital is a limited service small rural hospital that receives cost-based reimbursement for inpatient and outpatient care.

Diagnosis Related Group (DRG). A resource classification system that serves as the basis of the method for reimbursing hospitals based on the medical diagnosis for each patient. Hospitals receive a set payment amount determined in advance based on the length of time patients with a given diagnosis are likely to stay in the hospital. Also used as the basis of the Medicare inpatient PPS.

Direct Contracting. Refers to a direct contractual arrangement between an employer and a provider or provider organization for the provision of healthcare services. The two parties may negotiate rates for services in a variety of ways, such as discounted charges, per diem rates, or DRGs. Direct contracts may include use of third-party administrators for claims processing, utilization management, or other administrative functions. Direct contracting is often used as a cost-containment strategy since fewer costs are incurred by a middleman insurance company.

Durable Power of Attorney for Healthcare. Allows an individual to designate in advance another person to act on his or her behalf if he or she is unable to make a decision to accept, maintain, discontinue, or refuse any healthcare services.

Exclusive Provider Organization (EPO). A healthcare payment and delivery arrangement in which members must obtain all their care from doctors and hospitals within an established network. If members go outside, benefits are not payable.

Fiscal Intermediary (FI). An organization that contracts with the federal government to administer portions of the Medicare program.

Formulary. The list of prescription medications that may be dispensed by participating pharmacies without health plan authorization. The formulary is selected based on effectiveness of the drug as well as its cost. The physician is requested or required to use only formulary drugs unless there is a valid medical reason to use a nonformulary drug. Formularies may be open or closed. Closed formularies are restricted by the number and type of drugs included in the list.

Freestanding Ambulatory Surgery Center. A medical facility that provides surgical treatment on an outpatient basis only.

Full-Time Equivalent Personnel (FTEP). Refers to hospital employees; total FTE personnel is calculated by dividing the hospital's total number of paid hours by 2080, the number of annual paid hours for one full-time employee.

Gatekeeper. Term used to describe the coordination role of the primary care provider (PCP) who manages various components of a member's medical treatment, including all referrals for specialty care, ancillary services, durable medical equipment, and hospital services. The gatekeeper model is a popular cost-control component of many managed care plans because it requires a subscriber to first see their PCP and receive the PCP's approval before going to a specialist about a given medical condition (except for emergencies).

Health and Human Services (HHS). The U.S. Department of Health and Human Services, formerly the Department of Health, Education, and Welfare.

Health Insurance Purchasing Cooperative (HIPC). A large group of employers and individuals functioning as an insurance broker to purchase health coverage, certify health plans, manage premiums and enrollment, and provide consumers with buying information. Also called health insurance purchasing group, health plan purchasing cooperative, and health insurance purchasing corporation.

Health Maintenance Organization (HMO). A healthcare payment and delivery system involving networks of doctors and hospitals. Members must receive all their care from providers within the network.

- *Staff Model HMO.* Physicians are on the staff of the HMO and are usually paid a salary.
- *Group Model HMO.* The HMO rents the services of the physicians in a separate group practice and pays the group a per patient rate.
- *Network Model HMO.* The HMO contracts with two or more independent physician group practices to provide services and pays a fixed monthly fee per patient.

Health Plan Employer Data and Information Set (HEDIS). A standard data-reporting system developed in 1991 to measure the quality and performance of health plans. A main goal of HEDIS is to standardize health plan performance measures for consumers and payers. HEDIS concentrates on four aspects of healthcare: (1) quality, (2) access and patient satisfaction, (3) membership and utilization, and (4) finance. Within each focus area is a specific set of HEDIS data measures (e.g., number of immunizations for pediatric enrollees). The National Committee for Quality Assurance is responsible for coordinating HEDIS and making changes each year

Hospice. An organization that provides medical care and support services (such as pain and symptom management, counseling, and bereavement services) to terminally ill patients and their families. May be a freestanding facility; a unit of a hospital or other institution; or a separate program of a hospital, agency, or institution.

Hospitalists. A physician whose practice is caring for patients while in the hospital. A primary care physician (PCP) turns their patients over to a hospitalist, who becomes the physician of record and provides and directs the care of the patient while the patient is hospitalized and returns the patient to the PCP at the time of hospital discharge.

Hospital Market Basket. Components of the overall cost of hospital care.

Hospital Market Basket Index (HMBI). An inflationary measure of the cost of goods and services purchased by hospitals.

Hospital Preauthorization. A managed care technique in which the insured obtains permission from a managed care organization before entering the hospital for nonemergency care.

Independent Practice Association (IPA). A group of independent physicians who have formed an association as a separate legal entity for contracting purposes. IPA physician providers retain their individual practices, work in separate offices, continue to see their non-managed-care patients, and have the option to contract directly with managed care plans. A key advantage of the IPA arrangement is that it helps its members achieve some of the negotiating leverage of a large physician group practice with some degree of flexibility for each provider. Also referred to as independent physician association.

Integrated Care. A comprehensive spectrum of health services, from prevention through long-term care, provided via a single administrative entity and coordinated by a primary care gatekeeper.

Integrated Delivery Network or System (IDN or IDS). An entity (corporation, partnership, association, or other legal entity) that enters into arrangements with managed care organizations, employs or has contracts with providers, and agrees to provide or arrange for the provision of healthcare services to members covered by the managed care plan.

Joint Commission on Accreditation of Healthcare Organizations (JCAHO). The organization that evaluates and monitors the quality of care provided in hospitals based on standards established by JCAHO.

Length of Stay (LOS). The period of hospitalization as measured in days billed; average LOS is determined by discharge days divided by discharges.

Living Will. Document generated by a person for the purpose of providing guidance about the medical care to be provided if the person is unable to articulate those decisions (see Advance Directive).

Long-Term Care. A continuum of maintenance, custodial, and health services to the chronically ill, disabled, or mentally handicapped.

Magnetic Resonance Imaging (MRI). A noninvasive diagnostic technique used to create images of body tissue and monitor body chemistry. Uses radio and magnetic waves instead of radiation.

Managed Care. A term that applies to the integration of healthcare delivery and financing. It includes arrangements with providers to supply healthcare services to members, criteria for the selection of healthcare providers, significant financial incentives for members to use providers in the plan, and formal programs to monitor the amount of care and quality of services.

Managed Care Organization (MCO). A healthcare organization, such as a health maintenance organization, that manages or controls what it spends on healthcare by closely monitoring how doctors and other medical professionals treat patients.

Management Service Organization (MSO). An entity that provides practice management and other operational services to physicians, which can include facilitating managed care contracting.

Mandated Benefits. Certain services or benefits—such as prenatal care, mammography screening, and care for newborns—that states require insurers to include in health insurance policies. Sometimes called state mandates.

Medicaid. A federal public assistance program enacted into law on January 1, 1966, under Title XIX of the Social Security Act, to provide medical benefits to eligible low-income persons needing healthcare regardless of age. The program is administered and operated by the states, which receive federal matching funds to cover the costs of the program. States are required to include certain minimal services as mandated by the federal government but may include any additional services at their own expense.

Medical Loss Ratio. The ratio between the cost to deliver medical care and the amount of money that a plan receives. Insurance companies often have a medical loss ratio of 92 percent or more; tightly managed HMOs may have medical loss ratios of 75 to 85 percent, although the overhead (or administrative cost ratio) is concomitantly higher. The medical loss ratio is dependent on the amount of money brought in, as well as the cost of delivering care; thus, if the rates are too low, the ratio may be high, even though the actual cost of delivering care is not out of line.

Medicare. The federal program which provides healthcare to persons 65 years of age and older and to others entitled to Social Security benefits.

Medicare is administered at the federal level, as contrasted with Medicaid, which is administered by the states. Medicare was established in 1965 by amendment to the Social Security Act (Public Law 89-97), the main section of the amendment being "Title XVIII—Health Insurance for the Aged."

The Medicare program has been affected by a significant amount of federal legislation since its creation in 1965, including the Balanced Budget Act of 1997 (BBA), the Balanced Budget Refinement Act of 1999 (BBRA), and the Medicare, Medicaid and S-CHIP Benefits Improvement and Protection Act of 2000 (BIPA).

Medicare Geographic Classification Review Board. Five-person board, established by Congress in 1990, to review hospital requests for geographic reclassification for Medicare PPS purposes. To be reclassified, hospitals generally must be located in an adjacent county and pay wages equal to at least 85 percent of those paid by hospitals in the area for which reclassification is being requested.

Medicare Supplement Policy. A type of health insurance policy that provides benefits for services Medicare does not cover.

Medigap Insurance. A supplemental health insurance policy in which a Medicare beneficiary pays a monthly premium to cover the cost of health benefits that Medicare does not cover.

Morbidity. Incidence and severity of illness and accidents in a well-defined class or classes of individuals.

Mortality. Incidence of death in a well-defined class or classes of individuals.

Multihospital System. Two or more hospitals owned, leased, contract managed, or sponsored by a central organization; they can be either nonprofit or investor owned.

Neonatal. The part of an infant's life from the hour of birth through the first 27 days, 23 hours and 59 minutes; the infant is referred to as newborn throughout this period.

Nosocomial Infection. Infection acquired in a hospital.

Nuclear Medicine. The use of radioisotopes to study and treat disease, especially in the diagnostic area.

Nurse Practitioner (NP). A licensed nurse who has completed a nurse practitioner program at the master's or certificate level and is trained in providing primary care services. NPs are qualified to conduct expanded healthcare evaluations and decision making regarding patient care, including diagnosis, treatment, and prescriptions, sometimes under a physician's supervision; generally, they provide services at a lower cost than PCPs. NPs may also be trained in medical specialties, such as pediatrics, geriatrics, and midwifery. Legal regulations in some states prevent NPs from qualifying for direct Medicare and Medicaid reimbursement, writing prescriptions, and admitting patients to hospitals. Also called advance practice nurse (APN).

Nursing Levels of Education. The levels of education established for nursing are as follows:

- *LPN (licensed practical nurse)* — requires one year of formal training at a vocational or technical school
- *Diploma (RN)* — requires two to three years of education at a hospital school of nursing
- *Associate Degree (ADN)* — requires two years of education at a community college or university
- *Baccalaureate Degree (BSN)* — requires four academic years of education at a college or university
- *Master's Degree (MS or MSN)* — requires completion of at least one year of prescribed study beyond the baccalaureate degree

Open Panel. Allows for any willing provider to contract with an HMO providing the provider meets all the requirements set forth by the HMO.

Operating Margin. Margin of net patient care revenues in excess of operating expenses.

Out-of-Network Services. Healthcare services received by a plan member from a noncontracted provider. Reimbursement is usually lower when a member goes out of network. Other financial penalties may apply for out-of-network services.

Outcomes. The end result of medical care, as indicated by recovery, disability, functional status, mortality, morbidity, or patient satisfaction.

Outcomes Measurement. The process of systematically tracking a patient's clinical treatment and responses to that treatment using generally accepted outcomes measures or quality indicators such as mortality, morbidity, disability, functional status, recovery, and patient satisfaction. Such measures are considered by many healthcare researchers as the only valid way to determine the effectiveness of medical care.

Outpatient Care. Treatment provided to a patient who is not confined in a healthcare facility. Outpatient care includes services that do not require an overnight stay, such as emergency treatment, same-day surgery, outpatient diagnostic tests, and physician office visits. Also referred to as ambulatory care.

Over the Counter (OTC). Medicine that may be obtained without a written prescription from a physician.

Patient Days. Refers to each calendar day of care provided to a hospital inpatient under the terms of the patient's health plan, excluding the day of discharge. Patient days is a measure of institutional use and is usually stated as the accumulated total number of inpatients (excluding newborns) each day for a given reporting period, tallied at a specified time (like midnight) per 1,000 use rate, or patient days/1,000. Patient days are calculated by multiplying admissions by average length of stay.

Patient Satisfaction Survey. Questionnaire used to solicit the perceptions of plan enrollees/patients regarding how a health plan meets their medical needs and how the delivery of care is handled (e.g., waiting time, access to treatments).

Peer Review. An evaluation of the appropriateness, effectiveness, and efficiency of medical services ordered or performed by practicing physicians or professionals by other practicing physicians or clinical professionals. A peer review focuses on the quality of services that are performed by all health personnel involved in the delivery of the care under review and how appropriate the services are to meet the patients' needs.

Physician Hospital Organization (PHO). A type of integrated delivery system that links hospitals and a group of physicians for the purpose of contracting directly with employers and managed care organizations. A PHO is a legal entity that allows physicians to continue to their own practices and to see patients under the terms of a professional services agreement. This type of arrangement offers the opportunity to better market the services of both physicians and hospitals as a unified response to managed care.

Physicians Assistant (PA). A specially trained and licensed allied health professional who performs certain medical procedures previously reserved to the physician. PAs must practice under the supervision of a physician.

Point of Service. Members in a point of service HMO or PPO can go outside the network for care, but their copay and deductible will be more than if they had used providers who are part of the HMO, PPO, or health plan.

Point-of-Service (POS) Plan. A type of managed care plan that allows patients to choose how to receive services at the point when the services are needed. They may use out-of-network providers for an additional fee. Also called open-ended HMO, swing-out HMO, self-referral option, or multiple option plan.

Position Emission Tomography (PET). An imaging, technique that tracks metabolism and responses to therapy. Used in cardiology, neurology, and oncology; particularly effective in evaluating brain and nervous system disorders.

Practice Guidelines. Formal procedures and techniques for the treatment of specific medical conditions that assist physicians in achieving optimal results. Practice guidelines are developed by medical societies and medical research organizations, such as the American Medical Association and the Agency for Health Care Policy and Research, as well as many HMOs, insurers, and business coalitions. Practice guidelines serve as educational support for physicians and as quality assurance and accountability measures for managed care plans.

Preadmission Certification. Process in which a healthcare professional evaluates an attending physician's request for a patient's admission to a hospital by using established medical criteria.

Preferred Provider Organization (PPO). A plan that contracts with independent providers at a discount for services. Generally, the PPO's network of providers is limited in size. Patients usually have free choice to select other providers but are given strong financial incentives to select one of the designated preferred providers. Unlike an HMO, a PPO is not a prepaid plan but does use some utilization management techniques. PPO arrangements can be either insured or self-funded. An insurer-sponsored PPO combines a large network of providers, utilization management programs, administrative services, and healthcare insurance. A self-funded PPO generally excludes administrative and insurance services from the plan package. However, employers can purchase these services separately.

Primary Care Network (PCN). A group of PCPs who share the risk of providing care to members of a managed care plan. The PCP in a primary care network is accountable for the total healthcare services of a plan member, including referrals to specialists, supervision of the specialists' care, and hospitalization. Participating PCPs' services are covered by a monthly capitation payment to the PCN.

Prospective Payment System (PPS). Also called prospective pricing, a payment method in which the payment a hospital will receive for patient treatment is set up in advance. Hospitals keep the difference if they incur costs less than the fixed price in treating the patient, and they absorb any loss if their costs exceed the fixed price.

Provider Sponsored Organization (PSO). Public or private entities established or organized and operated by a health provider or a group of affiliated healthcare providers that provide a substantial proportion of services under the Medicare+Choice contract and share substantial financial risk.

Quality Assurance. Term that describes attempts by managed care organizations to measure and monitor the quality of care delivered.

Quality Improvement Organization (QIO). Federally funded physician organizations, under contract to the Department of Health and Human Services, that review quality of care and determine whether services are necessary and if payment should be made for care provided under the Medicare and Medicaid programs.

Reasonable and Customary Charge. Charge for healthcare that is consistent with the going rate or charge in a certain geographical area for identical or similar services. Also referred to as "customary, prevailing, and reasonable."

Relative Value Scale (RVS). A pricing system for physicians' services that assigns relative values to procedures based on a defined standard unit of measure, as defined in the CPT (current procedural terminology). RVS units are based on median charges by physicians. Physicians often use the RVS system as a guide in establishing fee schedules. This system is rapidly being replaced by RBRVS-based payment systems.

Resource-Based Relative Value Scale (RBRVS). A fee schedule used as the basis of the physician reimbursement system by Medicare. The RBRVS assigns relative values to each CPT (current procedural terminology) code for services on the basis of the resources related to the procedure rather than simply on the basis of historical trends. RBRVS includes 2,700 codes, covering 95 percent of Medicare-allowed charges.

Restricted Funds. Includes all hospital resources that are restricted to particular purposes by donors and other external authorities; the resources of these funds are not currently available for the financing of general operating activities but may be so used in the future when certain conditions and requirements are met. There are three types of restricted funds: (1) specific purpose, (2) plant replacement and expansion, and (3) endowment.

Seamless Care. The experience by patients of smooth and easy movement from one aspect of comprehensive healthcare to another, notable for the absence of red tape.

Single-Payer System. A financing system, such as Canada's in which a single entity—usually the government—pays for all covered healthcare services.

Skilled Nursing Facility (SNF). A facility, either freestanding or part of a hospital, that accepts patients in need of rehabilitation and medical care. To qualify for Medicare coverage, SNFs must be certified by Medicare and meet specific qualifications, including 24-hour nursing coverage and availability of physical, occupational, and speech therapies.

Surgicenter. A healthcare facility that is physically separate from a hospital and provides prescheduled surgical services on an outpatient basis, generally at a lower cost than inpatient hospital care. Also called a freestanding outpatient surgery center.

Swing Beds. Acute care hospital beds that can also be used for long-term care, depending on the needs of the patient and the community; only those hospitals with fewer than 100 beds and located in a rural community, where long-term care may be inaccessible, are eligible to have swing beds.

Teaching Hospitals. Hospitals that have an accredited medical residency training program and are typically affiliated with a medical school.

Tertiary Care. Refers to highly technical services for the patient who is in imminent danger of major disability or death.

Third-Party Administration (TPA). Administration of a group insurance plan by some person or firm other than the insurer or the policyholder.

Triage. Evaluation of patient conditions for urgency and seriousness and the establishment of a priority list to direct care and ensure the efficient use of medical and nursing staff and facilities. Triaging patients occurs in situations with multiple victims.

UB-92. The uniform billing claim form developed by CMS and used by hospitals across the nation to bill for services. Some managed care plans demand more detail than is available on the UB-92, requiring the hospitals to send additional itemized billing information.

Ultrasound. Refers to sound that has different velocities in tissues that differ in density and elasticity from others. This property permits the use of ultrasound in outlining the shape of various tissues and organs in the body.

Universal Access. The provision of coverage for healthcare services to all citizens.

Urgent Care. Care for injury, illness, or another type of condition (usually not life threatening) that should be treated within 24 hours. Also refers to after-hours care and to a health plan's classification of hospital admissions as urgent, semiurgent, or elective.

Utilization Review. An evaluation of the care and services that patients receive that is based on preestablished criteria and standards.

Wraparound Plan. Refers to insurance or health plan coverage for copays or deductibles that are not covered under a member's base plan. This is often used for Medicare.

Source: Iowa Hospital Association. 2003. "Healthcare Terms." [Online information; retrieved 6.9.03.] www.ihaonline.org/publications/termsweb .pdf.

About the Author

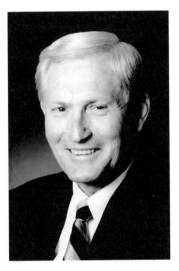

ERROL L. BIGGS, PH.D., FACHE, is the director of the graduate programs in health administration and the director for the Center for Health Administration, University of Colorado–Denver. Dr. Biggs received his PH.D. in health administration and planning from The Pennsylvania State University, his LL.B. (Law) degree from LaSalle Ext. University, and an M.B.A. in health administration from The George Washington University.

Currently, Dr. Biggs' primary research and consulting activities include work with hospitals to improve the governance of those organizations. He teaches governance in both the graduate on-campus and executive programs in health administration at the University of Colorado. He is also a faculty member of the American Governance & Leadership Group and chairman of the Practical Governance Group, both of which offer educational programs for hospital governing boards.

Dr. Biggs has been involved in both the investor-owned and nonprofit hospital industries, including 12 years as the CEO of large, teaching hospitals, and has directed the first merger of an osteopathic (D.O.) hospital and an allopathic (M.D.) hospital in the United States.

Additionally, he has served on several nonprofit and investor-owned boards of directors. He conducts seminars and retreats for hospital boards of directors, and is the author of several articles on governance. Dr. Biggs is also a coauthor of *Practical Governance* (Health Administration Press 2001).

Dr. Biggs is a Fellow of the American College of Healthcare Executives. He is also a member of the National Association of Corporate Directors, BoardSource, the Association of University Programs in Health Administration, and the Medical Group Management Association.

Dr. Biggs can be reached at 303/556-5845 or by e-mail at elbiggs@aol.com.

Additional resources from Health Administration Press

Executive Compensation
Guidelines for Healthcare Leaders and Trustees
Edited by Thomas P. Flannery, PH.D.

Healthcare executive compensation can be an intricate and difficult issue. How do trustees use compensation to recruit and retain top talent while remaining sensitive to the perceptions of their community? This guidebook addresses the many complex issues that must be considered when negotiating compensation packages. It offers advice on assessing leadership performance, income deferral strategies, executive employment contracts, and physician compensation. It also includes suggested public relations tactics that can minimize criticism of high executive pay in struggling healthcare organizations. Both for-profit and not-for-profit organizations are discussed.

Order No. BKCO-1154, $67
Hardbound, 311 pp, 2002
ISBN 1-56793-184-7
An ACHE Management Series Book

The Essential Guide to Managing Consultants:
Strategies for Healthcare Leaders
Michael E. Rindler

Should I hire a consultant? How do I select the right consultant? Get straightforward answers to your consulting questions. This quick, informative read will help you determine when to retain a consultant, how to select the best consultant for your situation, and how to work effectively with consultants. The book also provides numerous tools that will help you establish a productive relationship with consultants, including checklists for various consulting situations, sample requests for a proposal, and sample letters of engagement. Benefit from the author's insights gained over three decades of healthcare executive and consulting experience.

Order No. BKCO-1168, $61
Softbound, 281 pp, 2002
ISBN 1-56793-192-8

Prices are subject to change.

For quick and easy ordering, call the ACHE/HAP Order Fulfillment Center at (301) 362-6905. Order online at www.ache.org/hap.cfm.